The
Health Coach
Collective

Congrats on your Journey To Authentically Living Naturally

Powerful Tips to
Empower & Inspire
You to Live Healthy & Happy
Volume 1

Namaste' !!

From Visionary

Dr. Marsie Ross
The Self Care Crusader
Certified Integrative Nutrition Health Coach

Published EdLyn Press
Washington, DC

● ● ●

Table of Contents

The Health Coach Collective

The Health Coach Collective: Volume 1

Library of Congress Cataloging-in-
Publication Data is available upon request

ISBN 978-1-7341400-0-2

Printed in the United States of America

For your FREE Self-Care Guide visit
www.HealthyandHappyCoaching.com

**For information on how to
nourish and flourish**
www.EdLynEssentials.com

The Health Coach Collective

Powerful Tips to Empower & Inspire You to Live Healthy & Happy

Volume 1

Dedication

This book is dedicated to anyone who is ready to take control of their lives. We have all felt lost, broken, unloved or just beaten down at some point in our lives. But now is the time to get up and get moving past all the stuff keeping you bound! We came together to show you that you are never alone. We are here to empower and inspire you can keep pursuing your health and happiness.

With Love,
Dr. Marsie

From Visionary
Dr. Marsie Ross

The Battle For Control

It has taken me a very long time to realize that I have been in an abusive relationship. That may seem odd for some to comprehend because abuse, unlike love, does not feel good. But it's amazing how easily we can turn a blind eye to the "smack in the face" truth of reality. The telltale signs were there for years. Like most abusive things in our lives, it first starts off fun and lighthearted. The relationship brings comfort and security until it becomes a part of who you are. Then things change. As you start to understand the power that the relationship has over your life, you seek to be free. But your mind and body are not so willing to let go and allow you chart a new course. Unlike someone who has suffered abuse at the hands of another person, my abuse was self-inflicted, and my method of choice was food.

When I reflect on my early childhood, I understand clearly how my relationship with food started off unhealthy. I was born to a teenage mother who struggled to care for me. We were often hungry and living paycheck to paycheck, so our routine became feast or famine. When there was food, I often overate and overindulged in a subconscious way of preparing for the famine, which typically lasted until the next pay cycle. To make matters worse, when the refrigerator and food pantry were overflowing it was rarely with fresh fruits and veggies or whole foods. The low-income neighborhood where we lived did not have high end grocery stores with many of these offerings for our tight budget. Often the readily available foods were in boxes or in metal cans. So even in times of plenty the kinds of foods at my disposal did not change. As a child my favorite snack was butter toast with brown sugar on top. Although this high calorie and low nutrient treat was so bad for me it became a fond memory because it meant there was food in the house. As you can see, the relationship I had with food was rigged early to turn abusive!

Before my teenage years started, I went to live with my dad and "birthed from her heart" mom. My parents completely and undoubtedly changed the trajectory of my life. I went from being in an environment where teenage pregnancy, diabetes and obesity ran rampant to a loving home with structure and consistency. My father offered a strong role model for academic excellence while my mom became the steady stream of the unconditional love that I craved. We were the three musketeers!

My father was a stickler for homework and home cooked meals. Green leafy vegetables become a staple with every meal rather than a "special" occasion side dish. But even in this new healthy home, I still had the feast or famine mindset. At dinner, I would make what my mom called "man plates." My food was often piled high and spilling over. My mom would attribute it to my accelerated teenage metabolism although she still warned it wouldn't always be like that. I, however, knew it was more than metabolism. My internal survival instincts were still preparing for the famine. I did not connect food with nutrition or see the value in what it would do for my body.

As I grew up, the love, structure and stability my parents gave healed almost all of the scares from my early childhood. I graduated from high school, college and earned my doctorate in pharmacy. I was married before I was a mother, a homeowner and a professional. Being active was never a challenge. I love to exercise! I crave the heart pumping vigor that physical activity brings. As a result, I have none of the overt health issues that plague many of my

African American female counterparts, like obesity, high blood pressure or diabetes. I stand 5'8" tall so my height has given me some flexibility with how any extra weight shows up to the outside world. To hide the abuse and avoid making any changes in my mindset, I would use my love for exercise to keep an "I can just run it off" in the back of my mind.

I wasn't until I started my first company, EdLyn Essentials, that I realized that I did not know how to let food love me. EdLyn Essentials is a dietary supplement company with a mission to create products made with the highest quality of vitamins, minerals and herbal complexes. As a clinical pharmacist I grew frustrated with the supplements that included unwanted ingredients like red dye and fillers. This frustration lead to a full year of research on the extraordinary benefits of dietary supplements. I worked with a team who shared my passion for helping women get the nutrients missing from their food. But I quickly learned that before I could help anyone get what they needed, I had to first confront the demons that still lingered from my early childhood. It soon become crystal clear that I needed to evaluate and change how I related to food. Supplements should never be used as a quick fix or as a way to avoid eating foods that honor your body; yet for years this is what

I did. I would take appetite suppressants to control my cravings and lose weight instead of eating foods that nourished my body. But the time for allowing my past to control my future had come to an end.

During this time of reflection, here's what I learned about my relationship with food:

- I was addicted to sugar
- I often overate and overindulged
- I ate too fast and mindless
- I was dehydrated
- I had no idea what nutrients my body needed

And guess what? All of these traits started in my childhood. I was able to mask the abuse behind my physical fitness, height and clean bill of health but still, it was there. My relationship with food was unhealthy and more importantly, I did not have the tools to understand or appreciate the value that food was meant to bring. However, I did know that in order to have a loving and intentional relationship with food, I needed a clean slate.

In 2017 I enrolled in the Institute of Integrative Nutrition. I did this not to become a health coach, but to get the tools to face those demons head on! The yearlong program was life changing. I learned about macronutrients, micronutrients, the mind-gut connection, and so much more. But most importantly, I began the re-training process. With a childlike innocence I embraced learning about different foods and nutrients and how they relate to my gut, hormones, mood and brain function. In the process I also give myself the grace to make mistakes so that I could enjoy the discovery process.

If you're struggling with your relationship with food here is an exercise that may help you to begin your re-training process.

Ask yourself the following questions:

1. What is your first memory with food? Describe your eating habits from your childhood

2. How do you relate to food as an adult?

3. How has this relationship impacted your health and overall well-being?

4. How can you move from an abusive relationship to a loving and intentional relationship with food?

Change is hard but the benefits of what you'll learn about yourself will make it all worth it. Before I could make real change, I had to first purge my old way of relating to food. This is where you will begin your process. I've teamed up with dietician and Master of Nutrition, Jeanette Chandler, to create a 15-Day Restorative Detox. The detox is designed to help you release harmful toxins and begin the process of seeing food as a way to nourish and restore your body and mind so you can live with energy and clarity. As you walk through each day of the detox you will have the opportunity to reflect and journal. This part is critical because it will help you take control and your demons head on without fear.

So much of what shapes us as adults occurs when we are children and don't have the power to control our environments. As adults when we do finally have control of our choices, we often keep those same abusive habits and unhealthy mindsets that don't serve us. This book is here to give you the clean slate you desire and deserve so you can live healthy and happy!

About the Visionary

Dr. Marsie Ross empowers and educates women to take charge of their health & happiness. She works with women who are ready to get to the best part of healthy living so they can lead effectively, sustain quality relationships, and live with authentic confidence. As a mother, wife, and CEO, Dr. Marsie knows first-hand the uphill battles women face with supporting positive body images and maintaining good mental and emotional health. Dr. Marsie is a best-selling author and international speaker, Doctor of Pharmacy and Certified Integrative Nutrition Health Coach. Dr. Marsie is known as the "Self-Care Crusader." She is on a mission to build an army of self-care crusaders who embrace self-care without guilt or apology!

Healthy and Happy Coaching

www.HealthyandHappyCoaching.com

EdLyn Essentials www.EdLynEssentials.com

Booking Inquiries: ReadyToThrive@DrMarsie.com

Connect with Dr. Marsie (FaceBook, Instagram, Twitter)

@DrMarsie @EdLynEssentials

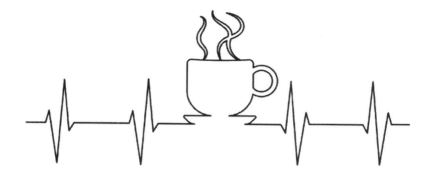

Unworthy No More!
By Anneka Davis, LMSW

The only person I've ever permitted myself to say no to was me. Sad realization, but it rings true for so many women. Growing up and even into my adulthood, I was overwhelmed by low self-esteem. I believed that saying no would hurt others. I wasn't aware of how deeply it was destroying me on the inside. I struggled for most of my life, not knowing how to take care of my mental and emotional well-being. I was starving for stability in my total wellness. I went to the gym, took excellent care of my skin, hair, feet, and nails; however, that was NOT self-care.

* * *

My emotional and mental self-care was disregarded. I was burnt out. I was stressed and felt very much alone. I suffered in silence for years, not knowing how to speak up for myself. I was yelling on the inside "STOP Anneka," but my world of pleasing others at the expense of myself just kept spinning. It was entirely out of control. I knew that there was something that I could do but was clueless on what that something was or how to execute it.

Avoiding putting myself first and moreover, not saying no when it was imperative to my survival to do so, caused me to become subjected to an abusive relationship for three years. I met a man I thought would soothe my soul and tend to the wounds of my heart. Instead, he tore my soul apart and depleted the last few beats of my heart that existed. When I met him, I was already in a very defenseless place. I had recently walked away from my five-year marriage with two young children in tow. Even in that relationship, I ignored all the signs that told me getting married was not a good decision. But I walked down that aisle and said yes, knowing that the answer should have been no.

After the divorce, the new man in my life took advantage of every vulnerability that existed in me. I hesitate even to say *"new"* relating its context to something "good," I thought, entering into a new relationship would contribute to my self-care. But the truth was, I didn't have an exact definition of what real self- care was.

Let me give you some background on what would become my downward spiral. When I left my husband, I owned my hair salon and spa. I spent a lot of late nights there. On one of those late nights, I met the man that could have been the cause of my untimely demise. You would think that owning a salon and spa would help me to curate a life of self-care. For me, it was what I could give to others but rarely partook in for myself.

I was too busy ensuring my guests had an extraordinary experience that left a lasting impression. Their self-care was my primary concern. I was consumed with providing happiness to others, and it was nonexistent in my own life. I masked my true happiness with this false idea that if others were happy, it made me happy. Does this sound familiar to you?

I was desperate for validation and "love." Like self-care, I didn't have a working definition of what love was or should be. So, I was looking for something that I didn't know how it was supposed to operate or what the exchange of it meant.

As I said, I stayed in this abusive relationship for three agonizing years. He began calling me names and cursed me out every chance he got. His words seared my low self-esteem.

For a woman who already had low self-esteem, it seemed nearly impossible that anything could burn what virtually didn't exist. The attacks then became emotional warfare, and that was where I started sinking deeper into one of the darkest places of my life.

My abuser was a pro at making me believe I was less than good enough. He told me things like my children didn't love me, my friends didn't respect me, and I didn't know what I was doing as a businesswoman. I began to question everything he said to me until it started to sink in and become a reality for me. He began to isolate me from my friends. He told me that my friends didn't respect me because they didn't support me in my business since they didn't do things like hand out flyers, spend late nights with me or come up with marketing ideas. I defended them because I didn't feel that it was their responsibility. He just called me stupid for thinking that way. He even tried to build a wedge between my children and me. I had to draw the line there.

My mental self-care was a blur. I was in a daze. My mind was flooded with ideas of unworthiness, fear, and the unwillingness to go on. Having two young children, there was still this protective barrier I attempted to build for them, but I somehow didn't have that for myself. He never made any verbal or physical attempts of abuse toward my children. If so, perhaps I'd be writing this from prison... if you know what I mean.

Yes, I allowed my abuser to have almost complete control over me. He controlled the way I spent my money, how I raised my children; he felt they should be more independent at three and nine, how I ran my business, who I should associate with, when I should call him and even when and how I should be intimate with him. An area that he tried but failed to take control of in my business with my guests or staff. Both groups would come to my defense when they saw how he was abusing me in front of them. My team would often hang up on him because of his incessant phone calls throughout the day. This would create and insight fear in me because I knew later that night, I would feel the brunt of his anger. Sometimes he would show up at the shop and interrupt my session with a guest or other work-related matters. They would always question what "someone like me was doing with someone like him."

How could I be in a place where I wasn't promoting my own mental and emotional self-care? I had a degree in Psychology and owned a business that focused on self-care for goodness sake. It was my mission to serve my guests with a dose of mental and physical wellness. I believed in providing a holistic approach to wellness and well-being. I played music that was relaxing, soothing, and calming. The décor represented the living room you desired you had at home.

It offered big comfy couches, soft lighting, aromatherapy, and the ability to do absolutely nothing for as long as you wanted. They also could confide in me as an outlet. They discussed many personal things that resulted in them gaining insight and peace. So where was the thrive, the push, the willingness to care for me, especially my safety and mental health?

I'll tell you where.

It was trapped in the belief that I didn't deserve it. My mind was warped. It developed this life of its own that told me that I could suppress the sadness, hurt, depression, and anxiety. Instead of addressing those things through self-love, such as setting myself as a priority, revealing my truth of living with abuse, tapping into the strength that lied deep within me, and setting boundaries, I chose to live in denial.

It took a lot of fight, drive, loss, and even homelessness before mental self-care kicked in. Enduring an abusive relationship isn't as easy as just leaving as most people who've never experienced it would believe. Most people say, "just leave"! However, they don't know that statistically, and for me realistically, the violence escalates, and even death occurs when the victim attempts to leave.

On a cold January night when I finally said enough to my abuser, he followed me to his basement, straddled me, and began to choke the life out of me while my four-year-old daughter laid on a couch sleeping just over my head. There was venom in his eyes, and I felt death enter my body. It seemed like an eternity that he had my neck in the vice grip of his hands. I tried to scream, cry out, plead, but nothing would come out. The only thing that appeared was a single tear, and suddenly it was over. He let me go. My head was spinning. I was dizzy, but I knew I had to run while I had the opportunity. It took me a few seconds to gather myself because I was nearly unconscious from him choking me. I grabbed a blanket for my daughter, who was only in her pajamas. I found a jacket for myself. I scooped my baby girl up and ran to my old, unreliable car and prayed it would start before he would catch up to us.

I was able to escape that night, but torture didn't end right away. I spent a while sleeping in my car with my young daughter. No one was aware of what was going on in my private life, so it took time before I opened up. I was finally able to speak out and reach out. I found a small place for us to live. Although I got away that night, I still wasn't free. He called me and followed me on numerous occasions. I was so fed up and tired of fighting for my mental wellness that one day I gave in. I attempted to take my life. I didn't want to die. I just didn't want to live that way anymore. At that moment, though, I heard God tell me to get up off the floor I was lying on and said to me, "That it was time to shift my mindset."

I knew that somewhere inside of me was a strong, powerful woman, but I knew to find her was going to be like digging in a gold mine. It was going to take so much work to shift my mindset and pour into an empty cup. I was dry inside. I felt like a plant that was still in a pot, but no one had watered it in forever, but it was still expected to grow. How could I dig that deep to save my mental wellness? I grew up watching my mother struggle with her mental illness my whole life. I desperately wanted to feel healthy, feel complete and whole, and know what it felt like to be in control of me. When you lack self-love and feel like your mental wellness is not intact, it causes you to make decisions that do not serve you well, especially when it comes to relationships. My mental self-care felt far out of reach.

So, the work to shift my mindset was slow and long but gratifying in the end. Enduring domestic violence breaks you in so many ways, so the work is continuous and repetitive. It requires much more than repeating affirmations to yourself, but it's an in-depth search in nakedness that helps to release the mindset shift.

Asking what the foundation is that allows an abusive relationship to exist is imperative to making the shift to mental wellness. If you continue to think the same, you'll do the same. I tapped into the things that allowed my relationship to exist. Not only was it low self-esteem, but it was also fear and unbelief. The fear was not thinking I was good enough for greatness. I also didn't believe greatness would ever exist in my life. I didn't believe I was great.

Shifting my viewpoint of myself was the initial work. I started to look into the window of my soul and began to wash out the dirt and grime that lived there. I was ready to eliminate that from my life. I scrubbed my mind of thinking negatively of myself.

When you remove something negative, it's crucial to replace it with something positive. I worked on ways to increase my self-awareness and how I was thinking about and talking to myself. Self-talk is an incredibly important conversation.

So, I was committed to positive communication. Self-care begins there. Of course, there were times negativity crept in, but I beat it down like a thief trying to rob me. There was no way I was going back down a path that would destroy my mental self-care or my self-confidence.

In 2010, I decided to go back to school to obtain my master's degree in social work. I was determined to learn more about how I could create and use methodologies that would increase my mental self-care as well as others. I no longer wanted to see women endure what I went through. For those that were already in it, I wanted to help them learn to shift their mindset to learn how to get out.

In 2015, as I continued to work in Social Services and define, redefine, and fine-tune my methods on shifting the mindset, I developed my business My Complete 180. I created a three-step strategy which is Admit, Assess, and Address to teach how to live a transformed life. I wanted to develop tools that would produce sustainable change. The work is challenging and sometimes painful. However, the rate of return is worth the investment. Making a 180 is not a one and done. There are always ways in which we need to and can shift our mindset.

Today, I continue to hone my craft and my methods. I also work on myself, as well. The mind can quickly revert to a more natural old way of thinking, and that is in the negative. Thinking positively is hard work, but it's worth the effort because the reward is a higher level of seeing yourself and being able to live a transformed life. We must pay attention to our mental self-care. As we check up on our physical health, we must put in the effort to check in our mental health as well.

I would tell women in an abusive relationship to consider seeking help. I know that it is challenging, but control, pain, and isolation is not love. Love does not hurt. 1 Corinthians 13:4-5 (NIV) reads; Love is patient, love is kind. It does not envy. It does not boast; it is not proud. It does not dishonor others; it is not self-seeking; it is not easily angered; it keeps no record of wrongs. We must love ourselves first to know that we should never allow harm to replace the true definition of love.

My three-step strategy toward sustainable change works in this way;

1. **Admit** that changing our mindset will free us from hurt, pain, and going down the wrong path.

2. **Assess** the steps that will be taken to make the sustainable mindset shift. Set attainable goals that will be accomplished in a measurable amount of time.

3. **Address** every single goal and maintain a level of focus that will assist you in making the transformation you set out in

the beginning once you've admitted that the mindset shift was necessary.

Loving yourself above all else will set you out on a path that will lead to success in all areas of your life. I believe when you set yourself as a priority, it is a reflection of positive mental self-care. Know that you are worthy, loveable, beautiful, capable, and fabulous!

ABOUT THE AUTHOR

Anneka Marie (A. Marie) Davis, LMSW is the Founder and CEO of My Complete 180. My Complete 180 is a Life Enhancement Network that provides the conversion tools needed to create sustainable life change.

Using her creative talents, educational background, and life experiences, A. Marie has nurtured My Complete 180 into a powerful resource to help other people navigate through the struggles and obstacles they face in their everyday lives.

A. Marie holds a master's degree in social work and has dual licensure in New York and Georgia as a Licensed Therapist. She has been coined The Mindset Coach for the work she has done in the Social Services and Coaching industries for the past 20 years.

As a survivor of Domestic Violence, A. Marie is dedicated to the advocacy, education, and volunteerism for other victims and survivors to prevent the occurrence of future acts of this type of violence.

In 2015, A. Marie was diagnosed with Trigeminal Neuralgia, a brain and facial pain disorder that affects the 5th cranial nerve. She has done extensive work to have the disorder recognized by the World Health Organization on its list of illnesses and bring about awareness to what has been described as the Suicide Disease, as 25% of those diagnosed commit suicide within the first six months of diagnosis due to the severe pain experienced. Although A. Marie has been impacted by the disorder, her drive and desire to positively transform the lives of those around her far supersedes her struggle.

It is the mission, passion, and desire of A. Marie to cultivate the shift of mindsets and the transformation of lives on a local, national, and international level.

For more information or to connect with A. Marie, visit her website: www.amariedavis.com.
You can also follow her on social media: IG & Linkedin @a.mariedavis and FB & Twitter @theamariedavis

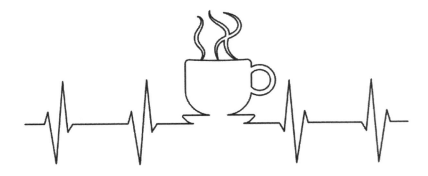

Rewriting Your Health Journey
By Ashley Murdock

I was sick and tired of being sick and tired. Not that I was physically sick, but I was tired of how I perceived my health and my happiness. I knew something needed to change. I began to reflect on various things that I have experienced in my life, and as a result, I decided to change my life and focus on my health. Trying new things, continuing my education, and having conversations with people helped me define what health means to me. Defining health on my terms in my own words was my biggest "AHA!" moment.

Being healthy means achieving wellness holistically across all aspects of life (mental, physical, financial, and spiritual). It means loving myself fully, being connected with myself and God, feeling excited about life when I wake up in the morning, getting energy from the food I eat and the workouts I complete and having money be a benefit and not a challenge.

I knew I wanted to live a life full of health, wealth, and happiness. To accomplish that I had to change how I took care of my mind, body, and heart, I had to shift from a mindset of restriction to liberation. I also had to challenge my beliefs and change my habits.

Now, I wake up in control of my destiny, my relationship with myself, and my relationship with food. Based on my journey, I have created a 5-step system that will guide you toward achieving a healthy lifestyle and developing healthy habits to maintain that lifestyle. But first, I want to talk about one of the most instrumental mindset shifts I had to make to begin elevating my health and wellness journey.

Mindset Shift: Having a Diet Mentality does not Lead to Lasting Change

I have tried every diet under the sun: the lemon pepper diet, protein shake diet, low carb diet, pescatarian diet, the list goes on and on. I believed that going on different diets would help me not only lose weight but also lead to my overall happiness and make me feel more comfortable in my skin. After going on all of these diets, the only thing I "lost" was my patience.

I always started each diet with the same goal, to lose weight and keep it off forever. The main problem with that was that I was expecting longevity from a quick fix. Let's be honest, diets are hard to stick to, and the majority of the time they lead to restriction, unhappiness, and weight gain. The word diet has the word die in it, and I took it literally.

My entire life would change when I went on a diet because I was restricting the food I was eating and my lifestyle. Each diet came with a laundry list of foods I had to give up and a strict schedule of how much I could eat and at what times. I found myself unable to attend work functions or go out with friends because I had no willpower and felt awkward about bringing my meal. Believe me, it was tough to pass up on open bars and free food, but I felt that if I didn't, I'd break whatever diet I was on. To make matters worse, every time I finished a diet, my cravings would take over, and I would revert to eating the same things I was eating before. Eventually, I would gain all of the weight back and then some.

The Whole30 diet was my last straw. On Day 5 of the diet, I caved and ordered a cheese enchilada platter for dinner. As I devoured my food, I realized that I had entered a vicious cycle that I desperately needed to get myself out of. Failing my last and final diet made me realize that dieting isn't the key to health. That's when I decided to make the shift from a diet mentality to a healthy lifestyle mentality. I began to work on myself holistically and develop healthy habits to lead to lasting change.

The Five Steps to Achieving a Healthy Lifestyle

These are the five steps that I have implemented to shift my mindset to a healthy lifestyle and to develop healthy habits.

Step 1: Redefine your definition of health

Most people think health is just about fitness and nutrition. However, health is more than just the food you eat and the workouts you complete. The World Health Organization (WHO) defines health as a "state of complete physical, mental, and social well-being." I break my health down into four areas of wellness: physical, mental, financial, and spiritual.

- *Physical:* This area focuses on the health of your body, which is determined by the food you eat, the amount of rest you get, and how you decide to move your body.
- *Mental:* This area focuses on your emotional, psychological, and social well-being, which is determined by how you see yourself and how you handle your emotions and interactions with others.
- *Financial:* This area focuses on the health of your finances, which is determined by your relationship with money, money management, and career choices.
- *Spiritual:* This area focuses on your connectedness to yourself, your belief system, and/or higher power, which is determined by your values, morals, and principles.

Step 2: Take a health assessment

Do you ever take time to reflect? To take an inventory of what you love about your life and what you want to change? To rate your satisfaction with different areas of your life?

Self-evaluation and self-discovery are crucial to growth. You have to understand where you came from and what changes have occurred or need to happen to get you to where you are going. After you have redefined your health, it is important to evaluate each area of wellness and identify what you are satisfied with and what you want to change.

Ask yourself the following questions and rate how you feel about each area of wellness by either marking the area as Unsatisfactory, Neutral, or Satisfactory:

- *Physical:* How do I feel about my current dietary and/or exercise habits?
- *Mental:* How do I feel about my overall mood, and how do I handle my emotions?
- *Financial:* How do I feel about my current financial situation?
- *Spiritual:* How do I feel about my connectedness to myself and/or a higher power?

Step 3: Create healthy habits

A habit is something you do consistently without even knowing you are doing it. It is a practice that is ingrained in your subconscious. The next step is for you to identify the habits you want to implement to achieve a healthy lifestyle. Look at your ratings from above and choose 1 or 2 areas you would like to change. Then, identify the healthy habits you want to adopt to make the changes. Ask yourself the following question to create a list of habits:

What consistent action steps do I need to take to change my physical, mental, spiritual, and/or financial wellness?

Step 4: Define both an ideal and realistic version of each habit

Have you ever told yourself that you were going to accomplish something, but then life got in the way? Sometimes that happens. You identify a specific habit you want to achieve such as working out five times a week, and all of a sudden that five turns into a two and you're beating yourself up because you didn't accomplish what you set out to achieve. Sound familiar?

When you are developing habits, it is important to further define each habit by identifying your "perfect world" version of that habit and your "life happens" version of that habit. The "perfect world" version of your habit is a goal you can achieve when your life goes exactly as planned. The "life happens" version of your habit is a goal you can achieve even if there are unpredicted changes to your routine or schedule. Having two different forms of habits creates the opportunity for you to achieve a healthy lifestyle regardless of what curve balls get thrown your way. Review your list of habits and create a "perfect world "version, and life happens version of each habit.

Consider the following statements:

- *"In a perfect world, if the stars were aligned and I have no interruptions to my schedule, I can achieve...."*
- *"If life happens and there are unpredictable circumstances that impact my schedule, I can achieve...."*

Step 5: Evaluate your commitments and priorities

Now that you have identified your healthy habits, you have to figure out how you can consistently accomplish them. You have to identify a way to make your habits a priority.

You can do that by reassessing your current priorities and commitments to determine which may need to be adjusted or removed to implement your new habits.

Ask yourself the following questions:

- *What habits are realistic to implement based on my current commitments and priorities?*
- *Are there currently any commitments or priorities that I'm willing to change to achieve optimal health?*

Case Study: My Own Health Assessment

Through this process, I identified areas of wellness that I needed to work on to achieve a healthy lifestyle. When I conducted my health assessment, I realized that I was not satisfied with my mental health, and I needed to change my relationship with myself. I also was not satisfied with my physical health, and I needed to change what food I was using to fuel my body.

Next, I developed a healthy habit for each area that was realistic based on my priorities and commitments. I'm going to walk you through my health assessment process for each area. I will also define my healthy habits and provide you with a couple of exercises and tips that you can implement as you define your health journey.

Mental Health Assessment

Name-calling is something I had a lot of experience within my childhood. Throughout life, I have been called "chubby," "porker," and my big brother's all-time favorite, "quarter pounder with cheese." Through the influences of bullying, mainstream media, and social media, I grew up and became a woman that had a hard time loving herself. I became my own worst enemy. Every time I would look into the mirror, I would find something to criticize, whether it was my "ham hock" arms, cellulite, love handles, thick thighs... I could go on and on. I would feel fat and uncomfortable in my skin. There were summers during college where I would never wear tank tops because I didn't want my arms to show. I would rather sweat profusely than look at my "ham hock" arms. I also owned a variety of Spanx that I would throw on every time I went to a party to give the illusion that I was skinny. It was my quick fix for the night to hide the features that I didn't like about myself. I had a hard time accepting and loving myself, and I thought the only way I could was by making a change. My problem was that my shift was fueled by hatred. I started dieting and working out because I hated my body.

What I needed to do was silence my inner critic and take steps to change how I saw and loved myself. Instead of using hate to fuel change, I began to use love to fuel my change. I started to work out because it brought me energy and happiness. I started making healthier food choices because the food provided me with nourishment, happiness, and comfort. I had to love myself enough to make a change. To get to this point, I had to speak to myself positively. I had to shift my negativity to positivity and work towards building a loving relationship with myself. I began to write affirmations to strengthen that relationship.

Habit: Affirmations

Affirmations inspire change, and they are a reminder to yourself of who you are and who you are meant to become. They are used to bring into existence what you would like to accomplish and how you would like life to be. Affirmations can be used as a motivational tool, a reminder, etc.

Perfect World Habit: To say affirmations daily
Life Happens Habit: To say affirmations on the weekends

Affirmation Exercise: Create a list of 3 affirmations for yourself. They can be across any and all areas of wellness. Begin your sentence with "I am so happy and grateful now" to further speak into your subconscious how you would like to feel and what you would like to experience.

My Affirmations:

"I am so happy and grateful now that I see the beauty in me. In my smile, my skin, my natural hair, my curves, and my mind."

"I am so happy and grateful now that I only shower myself with positivity every time I look in the mirror."

"I am so happy and grateful now that I have eliminated negativity, criticism, and self-hatred from my subconscious."

Physical Health Assessment

Coming from a diet mentality, I didn't have a good relationship with food. I would use dieting rules or cravings to control my eating choices instead of listening to my body. I would put restrictions on my food based on different dieting rules, and I had an "I can't" mindset. I can't eat that because it will make me fat, or this has too many carbs, or this has too much sugar. I also tended to veer off of every diet I tried because I had a sudden craving for Mexican food or fried chicken that had to be fulfilled immediately. "Food comas" were a daily occurrence because I would overstuff myself with food. My cravings were out of control as a result of my diet restrictions so I would eat food that didn't serve my body.

I had to press pause and start to get more in tune with my body and eat food that I enjoyed but also eat food that gave me the energy I needed to have a successful day. As I got more in tune with my body, I started to discover that my body did not agree with my fast food and eating out lifestyle. I also had to switch to an "I can" attitude to permit myself to experiment with different kinds of food to identify which foods serve my body and which foods do not. Food can feed you in a lot of different ways and should provide nourishment, happiness, energy, and comfort.

I started to realize that I needed to eat healthier, and that involved me experimenting with cooking my food. I learned about meal prepping and how I can make a variety of healthy foods that serve my body that can last throughout the week. Thus, I began to cook more and eventually came up with a meal prep routine that worked with my schedule.

Habit: Meal Prep

Meal Prepping is the process of preparing meals that can last for a certain amount of time. This allows you to remain in control of the food you are eating every day and minimizes the chances of you eating out because you already have food at home or at work with you. After a long day, you don't have to think about "what am I eating for dinner?" When you get home, you will already have a variety of options to choose from.

Perfect World Habit: Meal Prep every Sunday

Life Happens Habit: On Friday stock the freezer and fridge with healthy meals that take 30 minutes or less that I can make during the week (e.g., turkey burgers and sweet potato fries)

Meal Prep Exercise: Pick a day of the week and try meal prepping. Follow the tips and tricks below to help you get started.

Meal Prep Tips:

1. Schedule time to meal prep: Normally people block 2-3 hours on the weekend or during the week to meal prep. Sometimes they choose two meal prep days and cook for 90 minutes early in the week and then another 90 minutes in the middle of the week. I know this seems like a lot of time, but once you decide what works best for you then you begin to develop a routine, and eventually, you can decrease meal prep time to around 90 minutes total.

2. Plan your meals: Make a list of the meals that you want to cook. When choosing your meals, it is good to choose meals that have similar ingredients (e.g., vegan chili and vegetarian enchiladas). It's also good to select a mix of stovetop and oven cooked meals that way you can prepare multiple things at once.

3. Buy standard meal prep items: Ziploc bags are an essential item, and they can be used to season veggies and marinate proteins. Aluminum Foil is perfect to use for lining pans for meals that you cook in the oven, and food storage containers are necessary to separate and package meals.

Health is a Journey

By implementing this 5-step system, I have learned that your definition of health will continue to evolve as you progress on your journey of health and wellness. My journey has led me to use my experiences to help women develop healthy habits to achieve a healthy lifestyle. I have advised clients to utilize this system, and they have seen successful results. I encourage you to adopt these lifestyle changes if you are looking for similar results.

I'm excited to hear what you will learn about yourself and how you evolve as you go through this process. Please contact me at ashleymurdock@successfulinpink.com or @successfulinpink on Instagram and share your story!

ABOUT THE AUTHOR

Ashley Murdock is the creator of Successful in Pink, a health & wellness company that empowers women to live a healthy lifestyle. She received her Health Coach Certification from the Institute for Integrative Nutrition and has uplifted women through one-on-one coaching and speaking engagements at women's co-working spaces, workshops, wellness retreats, etc. She uses a holistic health approach to guide women through a journey that focuses on achieving wellness in all areas of life. She specializes in helping women improve their relationship with food, shift their financial mindset, practice self-love and self-care, and develop healthy habits to achieve a healthy lifestyle.

Contact Information

Successful in Pink

Email: ashleymurdock@successfulinpink.com

Phone: 323-717-2908

Website: www.successfulinpink.com

Instagram: @successfulinpink

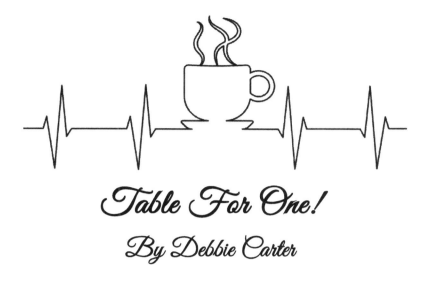

Table For One!
By Debbie Carter

I remember sitting in my walk-in closet, in a luxury 3- bedroom apartment I couldn't afford, facing the reality that divorce was imminent. I had tried all I could, done all I knew how to do, and cried repeatedly. This could not be my life. This was marriage number two, and I could not possibly fail at this thing again. The first time was to my high school sweetheart that I dated since age 15. He was the father of my children, and at the time, I loved everything about him. Fast forward to my mid-thirties, and I realized that this great man and awesome father, was not the husband I needed. We had grown into an amazing friendship, but the love was not there. Soon after, I was divorced for the first time and ready to live my life. The emotional pain from this divorce was absent for me because mentally, I had checked out of the marriage long before the paperwork was initiated. Or so, I thought.

Newly divorced and living on my own, I needed a part-time job to supplement my income, children's activities, and more. This is where I met my next long- term relationship. Attractive, physically fit, and did I say attractive. Yep, I was all in. All heart but little logic went into this relationship! He made my heart rate accelerate, and regardless of the red flags, I just had to have him. Yes, I knew his issues and shortcomings, but I am a fixer. Surely, I could fix this situation, and we can sail off into happiness. Less than a year after being married, I knew this was a mistake. In hindsight, he loved me to the best of his ability. I just needed more. By the time I realized that his best would not be enough, I was in my early forties, and felt my world was ending. How could I be divorced twice? Is this what my first husband felt when I announced I wanted out? What would my children think? Would God be disappointed in me? What will the family think? We just had an amazing wedding less than three years ago, and now everyone will know that I am divorcing, AGAIN!

Let me tell you how depression works. You wake and plaster on a smile when all you want to do is cry. You put on the fiercest clothes because you want your outside appearance to be the opposite of how you feel. When someone asks how you're doing, you say "I'm good," when in fact you are a mess internally. You shield your feelings from family for fear of judgment. After all, you are the family member that always has everything together. You put on a strong front for your children because you are their rock. There's no way they should shoulder your burdens. Your girlfriends are there, but do you become transparent with them? You may have one or two who genuinely loves you, but even then, you don't share everything you feel. So that leaves you and your thoughts. Those negative words that sound like, "you are unlovable," "no one wants you," "you are a failure," "you are in financial ruin." Yes, those thoughts consume you, and before you know it, you begin to believe it. Nothing but you and your thoughts running rampant. Slowly but surely, you begin to crumble.

In the midst of all of this, the one constant ray of sunshine was my weekly attendance at my local church. I was a member of a great church, with ladies who cared about my wellbeing. I attended weekly, looking sharp, and crying through the whole worship experience because that was all I could do to stop from breaking down. You see, strong women rarely break down in public. One Sunday, Rev. Dr. Ridley preached a sermon called, "One is a Whole Number." I remember her saying that the number one stands completely on its own. The number one is not broken or leaned to the side, but standing erect. That sermon resonated within me for weeks afterward.

I went on a business trip for seven days to Las Vegas. My good sister-friend would call this a "trip to the meadow." A trip away from everyone for self-reflection. You see I was broken and an incomplete woman. As I began researching the number one, I learned in numerology; the number one stresses self-sufficiency and self-determination. The number one represents the beginning of something new, a clean slate. The number one can only be divided by itself. I was the only thing holding me back. God sent me a reminder during these seven days of work and rest, mentally and physically, that despite all the "bad" in my life, I could have a clean slate.

I could stand tall, be self-sufficient, despite my period of brokenness. I had to begin to call a thing a thing — no more hiding. I had to file bankruptcy because I could not afford the financial mistakes of myself and my ex. But that was OK because I was on a journey to One. I had to break my lease and downsize to a one-bedroom. But that was OK because I was on a journey to One. I had to find out who Debbie was and remove myself from people for a while. But that was OK because I was on a journey to One. I had to stop emotionally eating and manage my stress because my blood pressure was dangerously high. But that was OK because I was on a journey to One. I had to find out what God's purpose and plan were for my life because for so long I was wife, mom, soror, daughter, sister, etc., but I had no clue what I even liked or wanted in life. I graduated from high school, had my daughter the next year, married two years after that, moved to a new state knowing no one, had another child soon after, and all along I was broken. Even after getting a divorce the first time and jumping into another long-term relationship that resulted in a second marriage, I still was broken and incomplete. I had no clue of who I was, so how could I expect my second husband or anyone to make me happy? I had to release all hurt, anger, and pain and look at me for answers.

I began a journey for self-love and self-awareness. The gym became my outlet, and there, I left all my worries

* * *

and cares. I dropped physical and mental weight. I changed my eating and became a vegetarian, the only one in my family. I cut my permed hair and went on a natural journey. I became aware of the energy I emitted and the energy of those I interacted with. For some, this meant I needed to limit my time with them due to their negativity. I took a journey of celibacy and decided that my walk with God was my focus and nothing else. I journaled and prayed. I got clarity and felt free. I learned that I loved morning walks and used that as a time to worship. I learned that while I can't swim a lick, being near water is my happy place. I learned that I could take myself on a date. Put on a cute outfit and ask for a table for one. I also told the host at restaurants not to stick me in a corner because I was not hiding my single outing. I learned to enjoy football and avidly watch my Steelers with pride. I learned to communicate better and listen attentively. I did spiritual gifts assessments and Meyers-Briggs assessments to learn more about my personality. I wanted to be a master of myself so that I could communicate with those around me how to best share my space. I did many things right, and some things wrong, but my period of self-discovery was essential.

In all my learning, I learned that leadership was my gift. My purpose and passion that would make room for my wealth. I learned about dominion, power, and authority from my current Pastor, Dr. Bradley. I learned that I am a child of God, and He has given me dominion over all things. I started getting ideas and words in the wee hours of the morning. I keep a journal nearby and could not sleep until I wrote down all that God was giving me. God was impregnating me with vision, and I was floored. Me?!? Do you know what I've been through? God, why would you want to use me? He answered by giving me words like healer- owner- inspire- empower, and more. I got visions of my future and was told a number of 38 million that I still don't know how that fits into my life.

At work, I managed a fairly large team. I had always been a problem solver. Things just come quickly and naturally to me. Where others sit and ponder over questions, I can quickly create a plan and implement it flawlessly. Coaching people is something I had done unofficially for years. I began to play around with a company name, logo, and brand. Based on issues within my own family, I also teetered on starting a nonprofit organization. After many months of back and forth, I decided to follow God's plan for my life. Doing it scared, I completed the IRS application for nonprofit 501(c)(3) status and launched 2Live Daily. Wouldn't you know it was on the same day that my long-standing stable job decided that they needed to downsize? Yes, add a lay-off to the list of things I dealt with. Welp, it was now just God and I walking boldly & authentically into his purpose for my life.

2Live Daily is a nonprofit organization focused on households of mental health patients. I work with this underserved population on networking, engaging in critical conversations, and equipping them with resources so they can make the best decisions needed for their households. I also coach individuals on finding, birthing & implementing their God-given purpose. I help organizations with solid business strategies to dominate their industry. I transform people and businesses from survival mode to a success story. I take average individuals and turn them into amazing stories of walking in power and authority. I show businesses how to lead their industry. I help people heal. I am a change agent. I am a walking testimony of God's goodness. I am doing everything God called me to do, and it is the scariest, yet most fulfilling role ever. God's word does not come back void. I am going to win because God said so. The timing is

His. The favor is His. The glory is His. I am because of Him. You will win because of Him. I am effective and thriving because of Him. My clients blossom because I am his vessel.

My journey for accepting my life for what it is and what it is becoming has been a process, not an overnight wake-up call. My process was about purpose, passion, and power. Every setback I experienced was a set up for God's favor in my life. I needed the experience of the divorce to learn humility and forgiveness. I needed bankruptcy to learn to be a good steward over what God has given me. I needed to isolate myself to be reminded that God is my provider, no one else. I needed to be hurt to understand God's, unconditional love. I needed to be laid off to wholeheartedly pursue what God's plan for my life was. I needed everything that happened because it was a part of God's plan and timing. Complaining about it gives the enemy a platform. Give the enemy an inch, and he'll try to take the whole thing. He's taken enough of my joy. What about you? Had enough yet?

Reader, I want you to be complete and whole not just for yourself, but for all relationships attached to you. If you are not complete, you are not useful to anyone. I encourage everyone to take a self-discovery trip, regardless of your marital status. It doesn't need to be in Vegas like my "trip to the meadow," but spend some time getting quiet. Learn yourself. Here's my assignment to you. Reflect on these questions. What do you like to do in your free time? What's your personality type? What's your love language? Where's your happy place? What's your favorite food? What's your favorite scent? Ever taken yourself on a date? Do you have a coach or mentor? What are you looking to "birth"? Why haven't you done it? What is holding you back?

How'd you do? Don't worry if you couldn't answer many of the questions. I'm only a call or email away to help guide your process,

Let me leave you with this: God is able. Years ago, I told God, if you send me another man, I'm going to need him to have this long list of qualities. If he doesn't have this laundry list of qualities, I don't want him. You see, searching for a man, AGAIN, was the LAST thing I wanted or needed. I was content in my space of One, and honestly, I still am.

Nope, I am not married again, but I am in the happiest relationship I could ever ask for. This man has

EVERYTHING on the list, except being a chef. He makes amazing reservations at top restaurants, though.

My closing tips: single readers, be a master of you. Go through the process of self-discovery. If it is in God's will, a man will find you while you are living your best life. Be patient and trust HIS process. At 49, and after two years of him pursuing me, I agreed to date exclusively. We have been connected at the hip ever since. For my married readers, make sure you are both whole. If not, it is not too late to stop leaning on another person and be self-sufficient. This is not about leaving your mate or suggesting you become independent. It is about being the best version of yourself so that you can spend your union complementing each other instead of trying to complete missing pieces of their life.

Finally, everyone should have a coach or mentor who pushes them to grow. Your coach or mentor should be transparent about their walk and use their life experiences to improve you. Good coaches and mentors have some education behind their business. They are also spiritually connected and can help you win at this game called life. That is your birthright and what God designed you for. Remember, one is a whole number. Stand tall. Coach Debbie

LeSean is rooting for you and available to help you grow through the process….

ABOUT THE AUTHOR

Debbie Carter is a certified Life Coach, Business Coach, and nonprofit owner. While going through a divorce many years ago, Debbie decided for business matters, not to use her legal last name. Instead, she uses the first and middle name given at birth: Debbie LeSean. A name she once despised is now her brand.

Debbie is focused on helping her clients flourish and thrive in life and business. Her assignment is to be a change agent to individuals who want to find, birth & implement their God-given purpose in life. She helps businesses with strategic solutions and leads a life-changing organization. Standing on Genesis 1:28, Debbie understands that all of God's children were designed to have dominion over everything they launch, create, touch, and govern. Her job is to reframe limiting beliefs, eliminate doubt, and provide customized techniques on how to win this game called life. Using her own experiences, counseling techniques, and outside of the box thinking, Debbie LeSean can help you find & dominate your niche in life.

Formally educated at VCU & Liberty University, and informally trained by the streets of the Bronx, Debbie credits the school of hard knocks as being her best teacher. The Psych classes, counseling courses, and executive leadership career experiences have been great, but God reminds her daily to walk it as she talks it, regarding her Christian journey and all things related to business practices.

Her nonprofit organization: 2Live Daily focuses on caregivers of mental health patients in educating and equipping them to make the best decisions needed for their households.

To contact Debbie call (804) 277-9069 or email: coach@debbielesean.com or visit her website www.debbielesean.com

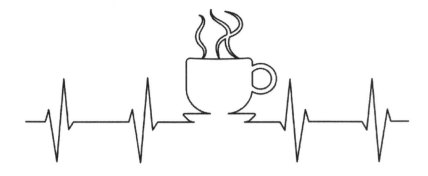

Beat the Belly Blues
By Jodi Jordan

I was about the age of seven; it was a routine child checkup at my pediatrician's office, the doctor plotted my height and weight on the growth chart and told my mother I was overweight. After leaving the doctor's office, my mom said to me, "don't worry; you're not overweight, you are just big-boned." For many years, I was the largest girl in my class. On multiple occasions, I was picked on for being fat. In today's world, we would call that bullying. Fortunately for me, those episodes were few and far between.

My diet growing up was filled with processed food and carbohydrates- frozen dinners, canned soups, fast food, pasta, potatoes, juices, and soda. In my middle school years, I used the Richard Simmon's Deal-A-Meal diet plan with my mom, who also struggles with obesity. This was somewhat successful. In my early teen years, I became more active and slimmed down to the point where I was happy with my body image.

My passion for helping others started early in life. I became an EMT at the age of 16, volunteering with my local fire department. As time went on the weight came back. At the age of 23, I graduated with my master's degree as a Physician Assistant. Topping out at a 200lbs, I had high blood pressure and refused to go on medication. I knew it was time to get serious about my health. I tried the fad diets, fat burner pills, the quick and easy, but never for any length of time as they often caused GI upset or made me too jittery. I joined Weight Watchers and successfully lost 40 lbs. If only I had a dollar for every snack and meal I've journaled in my lifetime. In the '90s, the thought process was to burn more calories than you take in, and you will lose weight.

To say I ate my share of convenient, highly processed 100 calorie snack packs is an understatement. As an oncology PA, working with cancer patients was one of the best parts of my career. I saw strength, motivation, hope, devastation, and plenty of death. Dealing with chronic illness and admitting patients to hospice was lifechanging. When you watch patients die, often at a young age, you realize just how short life is. I often need to remind myself…don't sweat the small stuff. Patients would say "live your life, don't wait until you retire; you may never get the chance." My husband and I began traveling, living life to the fullest.

I managed to keep most of my weight off, never required blood pressure medication and considered myself healthy except for heartburn and (self-diagnosed) IBS with chronic constipation. I was using Zantac daily to relieve my heartburn. My PA career took me into gastroenterology, department of corrections, and the military. To meet the fitness demands of the Army, I hired a personal trainer and learned how to do pushups, sit-ups, and eventually ran my first half marathon. Life was great. I had a supportive family, wonderful friends, a beautiful home, new cars, and the ability to take vacations several times per year.

Then it hit me; it was like a slap in the face. Looking back, hindsight is 20/20. The pieces of the puzzle start coming together. Twelve years into our marriage, my husband had become addicted to opioid pain medication and eventually moved to heroin. He would come home drunk or high, acting like a completely different person. I was scared; it was like living with a stranger. Outpatient drug rehabilitation and marriage counseling failed. Relationships with friends and family were destroyed, ultimately leading to divorce.

When someone has a problem, I want to help. I want to fix it. I want them to feel better. My therapist taught me to let go of the things I could not change. This was only the start of my wellness journey.

Through the divorce, I knew I was under stress, yet I didn't make the connection. The Zantac no longer helped my heartburn, so I moved onto Prilosec. I dropped to 135lbs, didn't smoke, and drank very little caffeine. At my lowest weight, I still had heartburn despite Prilosec and over the counter Mylanta. I took Prilosec every morning; sometimes it worked, other days, all someone needed to do was make a simple statement which gave me immediate heartburn or chest pain. This was how I discovered my mind-gut connection. I had the belly blues!

My support network was invaluable in the healing process. As the years went by, I remarried a wonderful lifelong friend and got called for my first deployment. I had been taking Prilosec for three years. Knowing medications can have long term effects, I reduced my refined carbohydrates, recognized when my heartburn was related to stress, and was able to wean myself off all GI medication before I deployed.

Spending 11 months away, I obtained my clinical aromatherapy and Integrative Nutrition Health Coaching certifications and Jodi's Wellness Ways, LLC was born. While I work with patients and clients on many different health issues, my passion is working with women suffering from obesity, IBS, healing the GI tract, and educating on the mind-gut connection.

Irritable bowel syndrome (IBS) is a functional GI disorder defined as recurrent abdominal pain or discomfort at least three days per month in the last three months with two or more symptoms of improvement after a bowel movement, often associated with a change in frequency or appearance of the stool (1). IBS has a constipation variant (IBS-C), diarrhea variant (IBS-D) and mixed IBS (IBS-M) where bowels alternate between both diarrhea and constipation. In functional disorders, all diagnostic imaging and workup are routine.

Functional GI and motility disorders are the most common GI disorders in the general population. Approximately 1 in 4 people in the U.S. have one of these disorders (2,3). The conditions account for about 40% of GI problems seen by doctors and therapists (3).

Note that IBS should not be confused with IBD. Inflammatory bowel disease (IBD) includes ulcerative colitis and Crohn's disease. In these disorders, there is an abnormal finding in the GI tract, often inflammation of the colon, ulceration, or bleeding. Bloodwork, x rays, and endoscopy can all be abnormal. Symptoms of rectal bleeding, weight loss, unexplained anemia, and family history of GI tract cancers are red flags and may require further testing by a physician.

Our digestive tract is quite complicated. Did you know that 80% of our immune system lives in the gut? Also, nearly 90% of serotonin, a neurotransmitter in the brain, "the happy hormone" is made in the GI tract (4). Serotonin plays a role in GI motility, sleep, appetite, and pain. IBS often coincides with disorders such as anxiety and depression. A frequent symptom of IBS is visceral hypersensitivity. This occurs when non-harmful stimuli are perceived as pain due to increased sensitivity of pain receptors in our GI tract (5). The nerve pathway between the brain and GI tract is often called the mind-gut connection, hence why the abdomen is also referred to as our "second brain."

Patients with visceral hypersensitivity report more pain than those who may have milder IBS symptoms. It is important to understand that an increase in abdominal pain often correlates with an increase in life stressors, lack of sleep, or even changes in diet.

While there are many different medications that can be used for IBS, I find that patients and clients do not want to take another pill. Once they understand what IBS is and what to expect, they often feel better with education alone. Reassurance is key. IBS is usually chronic, and symptoms can wax and wane during their lifetime. Dietary modification is of utmost importance, identifying triggers like refined carbohydrates, excess sugars, and processed foods. Patients typically respond well to a low FODMAP diet. However, it can be hard to follow. Low FODMAP (fermentable oligo-, di-, and monosaccharides and polyols) is the most common diet recommended for IBS. It includes avoiding high fructose corn syrup, excess sugars, artificial sweeteners and gas-producing foods like beans, onions, celery, carrots, apples, bananas, brussels sprouts, wheat, pretzels, bagels, alcohol, and caffeine (6). In the case of visceral hypersensitivity, you may experience more abdominal discomfort when consuming gas-producing foods (7).

There are many dietary theories. I encourage clients to make small changes and know that there is not one specific diet for everyone; this is the concept of bio-individuality. Clean eating is important. Stick to the perimeter of the grocery store focus on fresh fruits, vegetables, lean meats, and avoid processed or boxed foods. If the ingredients include chemicals you can't pronounce or don't know what they are, you should not be eating them. If our grandparents or great grandparents wouldn't recognize it as food, we shouldn't eat it. Our bodies also do not digest corn. In the US today, much of the corn is genetically modified and can cause GI distress.

Choosing an over the counter remedy for IBS can be overwhelming. Even before becoming an aromatherapist, I recommended herbal remedies to support digestion such as peppermint, fennel, and ginger. Ginger is perfect for nausea and has since become more readily available in the form of ginger root, candied ginger or ginger tea.

Fiber is helpful in both diarrhea and constipation but can contribute to gas and bloating. Probiotics, on the other hand, play a role in replacing altered gut flora with healthier bacteria. Probiotics often help relieve gas and bloating; however, they take 4-6 weeks for optimal effect. Physical activity is recommended for anyone with IBS and GI motility disorders. Walking and gentle exercise is important, especially when dealing with constipation.

I am very fortunate I chose a career that I love. Being a Physician Assistant and helping others is excellent. However, patients are becoming frustrated, being rushed through their doctor's offices, not having enough time with their medical provider, paying high copays for prescription medications only for pills to be ineffective or have side effects — This is what inspired me to become an aromatherapist and health coach.

One of my most memorable quotes from a former professor is "patients don't care how much you know until they know how much you care." As a practitioner, I don't always have the answer, but I genuinely do care. Patients are so grateful and appreciative of the time they spend with me as a clinician, and it's not because they leave with a prescription. I spend much of my day educating on IBS, the function of the GI tract, and the mind-gut connection.

As a health coach and aromatherapist, I work with clients alongside their physicians, focusing on the body as a whole, to make achievable, long term lifestyle changes so that they may live a healthier, happier life.

In closing, I've included some wellness tips and an essential oil blend to beat the belly blues.

Until next time, be mindful....be kind....be well!!

Health Tips

Drink water! As a rule, a healthy individual should drink half their weight in ounces. Adding fresh berries or fruit slices can vary the flavor. My favorite is adding a few slices of cucumber and fresh mint to my water bottle daily.

Chew your food well for better digestion, up to 30 times; proper chewing also helps release digestive enzymes to break down food, leaving you feeling better after a meal.

Eliminate pesticide consumption, opting for organic when possible – refer to Environmental Working Group (www.ewg.org) for your consumer's guide to the clean 15 and dirty dozen.

Decrease the use of plastics containing BPA's (Bisphenol A) & phthalates, which are linked to many health issues such as hormone imbalance, reproductive issues, and cancer.

Reduce your toxic load by considering natural beauty and cleaning products. Women are exposed to hundreds of chemicals per day in their beauty routine. It can take just 26 seconds for the skin to absorb harsh chemicals and hormone disrupters. Perfumes are among the worst. I like to add a few drops of my favorite essential oils to vanilla-infused jojoba instead.

Belly Blues Essential Oil Blend

Roman Chamomile (Chamomile nobile) is calming, great for the skin and a smooth muscle relaxant to help with digestion, stress, pain, and cramping (8).

Ginger (Zingiber officinale) is a warming oil, wonderful to combat nausea or vomiting and aides in relief of pain and spasm (9).

Sweet Orange (Citrus sinensis) calms anxiety, relieves IBS symptoms such as gas, constipation, cramps, nausea, and vomiting. Sweet Orange is also not phototoxic. (10).

Spearmint (Mentha spicata) eases muscle spasms, calms nausea, supports digestion, and eases pain (11).

2 drops of Roman Chamomile (Chamomile nobile)

3 drops of Ginger (Zingiber officinale)

4 drops of Sweet Orange (Citrus sinensis)

3 drops of Spearmint (Mentha spicata)

Add to 1 oz of your favorite carriers such as jojoba, fractionated coconut oil or unscented lotion and apply over the abdomen as needed for discomfort. A favorite carrier of mine is trauma oil, a blend of St. John's Wort, Calendula, and Arnica. This oil can even be used alone (without any essential oils) to help relieve sore muscles, pain, or cramping.

REFERENCES:

1. Lacy, B. E., Mearin, F., Chang, L., Chey, W. D., Lembo, A. J., Simren, M., & Spiller, R. (2016). Bowel Disorders. *Gastroenterology*, *150*(6), 1393-1407.e5. doi:10.1053/j.gastro.2016.02.031 Retrieved from https://wwww.uptodate.com

2. Talley, N. J. (2008). Functional gastrointestinal disorders as a public health problem. *Neurogastroenterology & Motility*, *20*(s1), 121-129. doi:10.1111/j.1365-2982.2008.01097.x Retrieved from https://wwww.uptodate.com

3. Parkman HP, Doma S. Importance of gastrointestinal motility disorders. Practical Gastroenterology. September 2006. Retrieved from https://wwww.uptodate.com

4. King, M. W. (n.d.). Biochemistry of Neurotransmitters and Nerve Transmission. Retrieved July 24, 2019, from http://themedicalbiochemistrypage.org/nerves.html#5ht.

5. Chiu, I. M., Von Hehn, C. A., & Woolf, C. J. (2012). Neurogenic inflammation and the peripheral nervous system in host defense and immunopathology. *Nature Neuroscience*, *15*(8), 1063-1067. doi:10.1038/nn.3144. Retrieved from https://www.empoweredautoimmune.com.

6. Hasler WL, Owyang C. Irritable bowel syndrome. In: Textbook of Gastroenterology, 4th ed, Yamada T (Ed), JB Lippincott, Philadelphia 2003. p.1817. Retrieved from https://www.uptodate.com/contents/treatment-of-irritable-bowel-syndrome-in-adults?source=history_widget

7. Zhu, Y., Zheng, X., Cong, Y., Chu, H., Fried, M., Dai, N., & Fox, M. (2013). Bloating and distention in irritable bowel syndrome: The role of gas production and visceral sensation after lactose ingestion in a population with lactase

deficiency. The American Journal of Gastroenterology, 108(9), 1516-1525. doi:10.1038/ajg.2013.198. Retrieved from https://www.uptodate.com/contents/treatment-of-irritable-bowel-syndrome-in-adults?source=history_widget

8. Butje, A. (n.d.). Login - Aromatherapy school and courses –
Aromahead Institute. Retrieved from https://www.aromahead.com/datasheet/data-sheet/aromatherapy-certification-program/chamomile-roman

9. Butje, A. (n.d.). Login - Aromatherapy school and courses –
Aromahead Institute. Retrieved from https://www.aromahead.com/datasheet/data-sheet/aromatherapy-certification-program/ginger

10. 13. Butje, A. (n.d.). Login - Aromatherapy school and courses –
Aromahead Institute. Retrieved from https://www.aromahead.com/datasheet/data-sheet/aromatherapy-certification-program/orange-sweet

11. Spearmint Oil. (n.d.). Retrieved from https://www.aromatics.com/products/spearmint-essential-oil

ABOUT THE AUTHOR

Born and raised in central Pennsylvania, Jodi Jordan is a physician assistant, certified clinical aromatherapist, integrative nutrition health coach, veteran and founder of Jodi's Wellness Ways, LLC. With 20 years of medical experience, utilizing both eastern and western medical modalities, Jodi works with clients to improve gut health and set achievable goals for a healthier lifestyle.

She also offers aromatherapy consultations and loves making safe, customized blends to help support sleep, anxiety, depression, gastrointestinal issues, and chronic pain. Services include health consultations, individual or group coaching and aromatherapy classes, corporate wellness packages, and speaking engagements. When not working, Jodi and her husband are often found seeking out new ventures in their RV. To contact or learn more about Jodi, visit:

Website: www.jodiswellnessways.com

Email: jodi@jodiswellnessways.com

Facebook: https://www.facebook.com/JodisWellnessWays

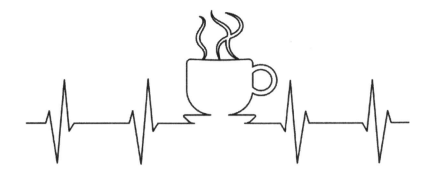

Authentically Living Natural
By Dr. La Tina Epps Thomas

Today, I loudly proclaim, I am authentically living naturally in my body, and I absolutely love me! I live my life, knowing who I am and Whose I am. I unapologetically keep what serves me well and remove what doesn't. I know without a shadow of a doubt, I deserve the very best from my myself, the people in my life, the food I eat, and anything else that is a part of my journey because I am worthy of the very best.

Bold statements, aren't they? Not only can I say these things, I mean them. Can you do the same? If not, you're not alone, but you can. For it wasn't that long ago I too couldn't think like this, let alone say it. I didn't get to this point in my life until I was so broken down that I had nothing left. I was completely mentally, physically, and emotionally beat down.

I was 35lbs overweight, depressed, and physically sick all the time. My mind was completely scattered, and I couldn't remember anything.

To the outside world, I seemed to be living a charmed life as if I had it all together. I was teaching several successful yoga classes and had some high-profile private yoga clients that I taught weekly. I was facilitating numerous stress reduction workshops for various corporations. I was involved in several civic organizations, actively involved in my church, and always showed up and tried to do the most to make everyone happy. I tried to be the best daughter, wife, and friend that anyone could ask for. I tried everything I could to be the perfect people pleaser, to not disappoint anyone.

Sound familiar? The truth is, I was living an inauthentic lie. I hated myself, I hated what my life had become, and I had no hope. What nobody knew was, the only thing that stopped me from committing suicide was the thought that it would kill my parents, and the people pleaser in me just couldn't hurt them like that.

I'm sure your thinking, didn't she just say, she is authentically living naturally in her body, and she absolutely loves herself? I did. So, let me start from an earlier part of my journey.

Remember, this life is a journey and as Judith Hanson Lasater, Ph.D., P.T. says, "everyone has to go through the woods and meet the Big Bad Wolf to get to Grandma's house."

My health quest goes back a few years to when I was in high school. In the not so long ago past (ok it's been a while, but I'm not counting!) A group of my friends and I decided we wanted to lose weight. To accomplish this, with our infinite wisdom as teenagers, we determined we would starve ourselves to do it! It just so happened, that at that time our peer counseling group, actually led by me, had a week on topics dealing with various stressors for a teenager. One of the videos that were shown was on eating disorders! Instead of being a deterrent for me, it became my bible! I took notes on everything you were not supposed to do so that

I could turn around and be the perfect anorexic! It's harder than you think. When I realized I was hungry, I added to my tactics. I would gorge myself! Of course, that was not going to get me skinny, so I took on the role of bulimic as well. On the occasion when my body couldn't function anymore on diet coke and 1 or 2 snack cakes or a small salad, I would gorge and eat everything in sight! Then I would feel so guilty and out of control that I would purge! Thus, began a lifetime of food issues, yo-yo diets, and the pursuit of becoming the best anorexic/bulimic I could be. At one point, my mom found me vomiting up blood. This led to me being hospitalized for ten days because I had severely damaged my esophagus. Go figure.

I'm sure some of you are thinking, where were my parents? How could they have possibly not known? Well, it was easy. I hid it very well. Remember, I was the ultimate people pleaser. I was the model child. I was into every activity possible. The French club, show choir, theatre and drama club, student council, and I started the Peer Counseling group in my school. I took all AP classes and worked hard to get excellent grades. I was friends with the popular crowd, the athletes, the druggies, and the nerds! I was that overachiever trying to be perfect at everything girl.

And my biggest fear was disappointing my parents. Yet, even after all the activities, excellent grades, etc. I never felt pretty enough or smart enough or popular enough! I never felt like I fit in. I didn't look like the pretty girls in my high school. You see, I was the only person of color in my all-white small-town high school in rural Wisconsin. Quite frankly, I didn't realize until a few years ago, how much that actually affected me.

My parents weren't divorced; they were incredibly supportive of everything I did or wanted to do! They told me I was beautiful and intelligent and could do anything I set my mind to. They taught me as a biracial woman to celebrate both sides of my ethnicity; it made me special. But in the process, that specialness had me feeling like I had a spotlight on me all the time. Especially when during sophomore year social studies, when the teacher showed the movie Roots to talk about slavery. This was the only thing discussed regarding Black people. They never taught that Black people were Kings and Queens. They had discovered language, technology, science. In fact, many of these things we are still trying to understand today. All we saw were black people as slaves, being beaten, raped, sold, and killed. My parents did do an excellent job of teaching me the story of Black people before slavery. But let's face it when you're a teenager in a high school where no one else looks like you, you feel the weight of the entire Black culture on your shoulders.

As amazing as my parents are, they weren't perfect. My dad had a tendency of buying me lots of things whether they were necessary or not, to compensate for the fact that he was gone a lot working. This taught me, as long as someone buys you expensive things, then they love you. It doesn't matter if your need for attention or affection is met. It also taught me that I shouldn't complain or speak up or want more because I wouldn't get those material things and in turn wouldn't be loved. My mom did the very best she could to mitigate those feelings.

At some point, my parents noticed something was wrong with my self-esteem. I was really hard on myself, even though to the outside world, I was outgoing and charismatic. It looked like I had it all together, but clearly, I didn't. Notice a pattern? So, they put me into modeling because they thought that would help. Modeling just put me into contact with lots of girls who had perfected the eating disorders game.

It made me a "professional" anorexic/bulimic. I truly believed that if I were thinner, I would fit in and be all those things my parents and family said I was. I would be in control. And on the days when I would eat only an apple and a snack cake, and I was able to fight the horrible gnawing hunger inside me, I felt invincible. Like I had everything under control. Instead, I was so far from being in control. My food issues were ultimately in control, and I was literally killing myself because of the stress and the eating choices I was making!

This is how my lifelong journey of food issues and low self-esteem began. A few years after college, I had an amazing career working in sports and entertainment marketing in a large major city. I had the opportunity to experience things that most people will never get to experience. But my low self-esteem and unhealthy lessons I learned as a child, lead me to make unsafe and unwise choices. I eventually lost everything, including my job and my home. I was homeless living out of my car and extended stay hotels for a few days. I couldn't call my parents or tell anyone and risk disappointing them, by letting them know I wasn't still living this "charmed" life. My homelessness didn't last long, however. I ultimately broke down, called a friend, and moved in with her. When I eventually called my parents, I ended up moving to another state to live with my dad. I was burnt out, depressed, and at what I thought was the lowest point in my life. But it wasn't because I hadn't learned my lesson yet. I still hadn't learned who I was or Whose I was. I hadn't learned that to live in my body truly; I had to rely on The Creator for my strength and happiness. That only He could fill that hole that lived inside of me. That hole of self-doubt and lack of self-worth. That hole that seemed as vast as the oceans. I hadn't learned how to authentically live natural.

My journey came to a head a few years later, when to the outside world, I once again looked like I was living this charmed, amazing life. I was living all of the things I talked about in the beginning. But in reality, I was beaten down physically, emotionally, and mentally. I ended up going to stay with my parents for a few months to help my mom take care of my aunt. Soon after I got there, my furry baby Max ran away. We spent five desperate hours looking for him. When I couldn't find him, I broke down sobbing uncontrollably. Everything inside me was done. I literally couldn't take anymore and felt like I was losing my mind. All I wanted was to be out of this pain. I wanted out of this life. I could hear my parents debating whether they should have me committed or not.

I was having a nervous breakdown. I went to my room, laid down, and started laughing. That's when I told God I give up. I'm done. I don't care anymore and that I give up trying to control anything. At that moment, the house became very quiet and very still. A few minutes later, I heard a meow outside the back door. God brought Max home. Then I heard Him say, "Now watch Me work!"

That is when the real work began. Lessons that I learned that you could incorporate into your life too.

I started by finding an amazing counselor and going to counseling sessions twice a week. I encourage you to do that if you find yourself with feelings of overwhelming depression or suicidal thoughts. We need to get over the idea that going to a professional counselor is a bad thing or is unchristian. Just like God made multiple other kinds of doctors for various issues, God made professional counselors too.

I then consciously made a decision that I was going to make a change. I started saying this prayer every day, which I still do to this day.

Lord, please...............

Help me to see my beauty the way You see my beauty.

Help me to see my intelligence the way You see my intelligence.

Help me to see my body the way You see my body.

Help me to see my worth the way You see my worth.

And Help me to love myself the way You love me.

This is really powerful. And you know what? He did! You see, the way you're living in your body now is exactly what will create the body you'll be living in in your future. The attitude, the beliefs, and emotions of today literally manifest in the form of your future body...whether bigger or smaller, more or less energetic, more or less healthy.

The easiest way to understand this is to actively and consciously do things that put you directly in you're here and now experience of life as often as you possibly can. Begin to recognize fully "all the things you don't want" in your life and for your body, and then re-frame these things and begin to create new ones, so that later you can create and sustain what you really **_do_** want.

I do this by participating in things regularly that support and remind me of what I want to bring into being. I started by first exploring some things about myself and my thoughts about my body. I want you to answer these questions and be truthful with yourself.

- Are you truly living in your body today? If so, how?

- Are you waiting for something to be better?

- Do you live in your body from a place of not good enough, not thin enough, not healthy enough, not strong enough?

- What things could you do in your life RIGHT NOW to remind you to be fully who you are?

What things could you do that remind you to live in your body EXACTLY as it is today?

Whatever you may or may not like about your body, it is the beautiful, amazing temple that God made in His image!

Here's the thing, when you do things that help you to remember how wonderful it is, guess what? You start doing more and more (and the doing becomes easy) of the things you know are good for your body. So, how can you begin to learn what is good for your body?

- Choose a few interesting simple things that speak to you and try them out. Like a healthy cooking class or horseback riding or yoga!

- Choose foods that make you feel alive and healthy and strong!

- Choose things that feel like, yes, I can live in my body and my life more when I do this.

- If you don't know for sure what those things are, experiment and have some fun.

AND HERE IS THE REAL KEY:

- If it's not fun, don't do it! Try something else. You're not a tree! Move on!

I lived a very long time thinking that if I were just thinner, I would be prettier, my boyfriend wouldn't cheat on me, I would be more confident, etc. The problem was, none of those issues had anything to do with weight or size. When I was in the height of my eating challenges, I was incredibly thin, yet I still had the same problems and felt the same way! Those were all self-esteem issues and by-products of me not fully loving myself or living authentically in my body. I was allowing my body to become a source of pain, not strength, fun, and adventures.

You can change this thinking. Here are a few simple ways how:

Stop apologizing.

This is extremely important. Stop apologizing to others for yourself. Save your apologies for the very few times they are called for in your life. Set the intention to stop the things you say both to yourself and out loud that carry apologies that diminish you. Apologizing is sometimes a subtle way we minimize ourselves, our value, and our power.

Whatever the current state of your mind or body right now, or how you're living in it, you've arrived here for a reason. Every judgment and every extra pound, real or imagined. Now, it's time to recognize the pattern and change it and stop apologizing for it!

Stop postponing feeling good.

The habit of "I'll let myself feel good when..." is destructive. This is a kind of holding out on yourself; it erodes the self-supportive you and leaves no space for you to grow your self-trust and your intuition. Stop trying to teach yourself a lesson.

For example, if you think you ate too much for dinner two nights in a row, it doesn't mean you've failed, or that you should give up on your intention to eat lighter meals. It just means going forward you eat smaller meals. That would be like if you dropped a hundred-dollar bill yesterday, and you decide you were going to throw the rest of your money away today! Does this make any sense? Nope.

Sit down and start a running list of simple things that you KNOW make you feel good.

Keep it with you so you can add to it whenever you have a chance. When you DO feel good, check and see what contributed to those feelings? Was it something you ate? Something you did? Something you said?

Stop being so nice.

A lot of times, we use our sweetness or our niceness to compensate for what we think is wrong with us or our bodies. This is related to stop apologizing or accommodating when we don't authentically feel like it. A distinct way to know if you're doing this is to ask yourself, "Would I be acting this way right now if I felt great inside and about myself and my body?" What I'm saying is, make sure your sweetness is real and your niceness is genuine.

Step out and have fun!

One of the most powerful ways I know to start honoring your body exactly as it is right now is to own your fun with it. Go out and play. Swing on a swing, run down a hill, go bike riding. I'm not sure who they are, that said as we get older, we have to stop playing, but they lied! Go out and play and have some fun.

By utilizing these and other principles, I lost 35lbs. More importantly, I now love how my body feels, and I choose to eat foods that help me maintain this strong and healthy feeling that I have. This doesn't mean I don't occasionally eat tacos, pizza, or a piece of chocolate. I don't eat a lot of it. I don't NEED to eat them. I CHOOSE to eat them.

This has spilled over to every part of my life! I choose to do things that serve me well. I choose the right to say no, or I can't and be entirely ok with it. I now realize I have to be true to me and how I honestly feel. This is the only way to authentically live naturally in the beautiful body that I have.

The exciting part is, you too can change the way you feel about your journey and live a life expecting the very best from yourself, from the people in your life, and from the food that you eat because you are worthy of the best. And you don't have to do it alone. I can help you, regardless of what your journey has looked like up to now.

Remember you're not a tree, you can move. Right now, today you can choose the path to truly authentically living naturally in your body, OR you can choose to stay on the course you're on.

As for me, I chose how I was going to live in my body, and today; I loudly proclaim, I am authentically living naturally in my body, and I absolutely love me! What will you choose?

ABOUT THE AUTHOR

LaTina Epps Thomas, ND, EYT is a Naturopathic Doctor, Experienced Certified Yoga Teacher, Corporate Health and Wellness Educator, Writer and Public Speaker. She is the founder of Authentically Living Natural, successful practice in Memphis, TN. She thrives on using her skills to help support bodies to heal, while also bringing balance and connectivity to lives.

Dr. LaTina has garnered acclaim for her success in helping numerous athletes and clients achieve their health goals through healthy lifestyle changes and yoga. Her passion for helping others stems from her struggle with an eating disorder. As a teenager, she fought a long battle with anorexia/bulimia. She won by changing her mindset about herself and food while incorporating the healing benefits of yoga. This put her on a path to better health and healing for herself and countless others. Today, Dr. LaTina is a highly sought-after instructor and speaker by numerous fortune 500 companies, while running a thriving telehealth practice.

When not practicing yoga or making herbal concoctions, Dr. LaTina enjoys traveling the world with her husband and relaxing with her two furry babies Kitty and Max.

Naturopathic Doctor, Experienced Certified Yoga Instructor and *a Health and Wellness*
La Tina Epps Thomas, ND, EYT
www.alnhealthandwellness.com
901-494-4579
drthomas@alnhealthandwellness.com
FaceBook: @alnhealthandwellness
Instagram: latina_thomas
Twitter: alnhealth
Linkedin: La Tina Epps Thomas, ND
YouTube: ALN Health and Wellness TV
Publicist: DC Cole – 214-680-5599; ddc22@aol.com

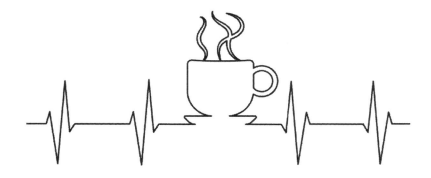

Releasing the Superwoman Mentality
By Coach Melody McClellan

SU-PER-WOM-AN definition, a woman with exceptional strength or ability, especially one who successfully manages a home, raises the children, and has a full-time job. Before we begin, Coach Melody's definition of a super-woman having to juggle it all, family, work, home, career, activities, appointments, caregiving and any other situation in your life. I know how important these obligations are, but I want to focus on you right now. Imagine what it would feel like taking one or two things off your to-do list and replace that action with 30 minutes for yourself. Fact, our country is experiencing a health epidemic with stress, heart disease, diabetes, hypertension, obesity, and the various forms of cancer. I am convinced from my research that many of these can be eliminated by lightening your load of responsibility. We all have 24 hours in a day and a choice of what to do with them. What are you choosing to make a priority with your time? Let this be an "AHA" moment for you. I have worked with countless women and been the women with the title of superwoman without thinking about it. Once you have identified this syndrome, it is time to make some changes. I use this saying, "when you know better you do better." I will use myself as an example, early on in my optimistic mind, I imagined I could take it all on, including marriage, kids, work, social life, activities, and it would be perfect. Yes, quickly, I learned balance was needed, and I had to prioritize myself. I started with a schedule that included me, but sometimes everything was not always immaculate or perfect. My thought process had to change to find peace and decrease stress. This helped me maintain my sanity. My motto is; "If it can't get done today, there is always tomorrow." Adopt some rituals that are centered and about you. Be unapologetic about taking time for yourself. I often hear from clients and people, "I do not have time." People make time for things and people who are important to them. Are you important to you?

30 Minutes To Start…You Are Worth It

Start with small, simple changes. For example, adopt one or two daily rituals that include yourself starting with only 30 minutes. Think of this as an investment in yourself begin with a plan and set S.M.A.R.T. goals (Specific, Measurable, Attainable, Realistic, Timely) you wish to accomplish then implement 1 or 2 goals each week, overtime these will add up. Remember this is about lifestyle change so DO NOT take on too much otherwise the superwoman mentality will begin to set in. You must take control, which is a habit that will take time to break, but you can do it! Create a healthy regime; I recommend you find a time that fits into your schedule and practice it daily. It takes time to develop the habit, but with consistency and goals it will become second nature. It is crucial to adopt a new mindset and create an effective plan which will take discipline but fundamental to your success. If you are one that stays up all night working, cleaning, laundry, social media, watching tv, STOP, the list is there waiting for you the next day. Proper rest and uninterrupted sleep are important to your body being able to reset and restore itself. The amount of time for adequate rest varies but typically 7 to 9 hours is recommended. This will allow you to wake up refreshed and energized to take on all the duties of the day. Make sure you are listening to your body, which will help reduce stress. It is easy to have stress and not know, especially if it is internal. If it is manifesting internally, your body can be thrown off sync.

Stress is known to be associated with autoimmune diseases. Some natural stress relievers meditating, yoga, reading, journaling any mindless activity. Do not forget physical activity is an option for stress release, like walking, riding your bike, swimming, dancing, and massages.

Write down what you enjoy? Whatever that is, I want you to take time and incorporate in your 30 minutes whatever pleases you. Keep in mind you can always break up the 30 minutes. No matter what, make it a priority to destress, this will keep you upbeat and in a good mood. Why am I telling you this? As a Certified Holistic Health Practitioner, I work with various women in the workplace and privately, and I hear this over and over. "I am taking care of everyone else and leaving me out." Women, by nature, are created to care for others, and that is ok. You also have to care for yourself. I promise once you incorporate the 30 minutes, you will begin to look forward to it, and you will never return to the superwomen mentality.

By no means am I suggesting you to not take care of your home, families, work, or any other obligations, just be sure to fit yourself in daily. You can invest 30 minutes out of 24 hours. Right? Create a healthy eating regime this is important because food is fuel for your body to run. Just like your vehicle will not move on empty, neither will your body if you are not taking proper care of it. Eat right, exercise, sleep, and get some self-care this is my secret for having peace in your life. No need to be a superwoman all the time. When thinking about health, wellness, and my "message," I consistently return to my saying, "Always invest in your health." You only get one life, take care of yourself before it is too late. As women, way too often, we neglect to feed our body, mind, and soul with what is needed to be present, vibrant, and whole. There is no better time than now to focus on self.

Coach Melody's Truth

I have written this chapter to be vulnerable and transparent, letting readers know it can happen to anyone. How, do you ask? I am a wife, mother, managed a corporate career, church, sorority, home, kids schedule, and other activities and responsibilities. Guess what happened, my body slowed me down cold. Interesting because I would tell others my career and life was high energy, which began to manifest as stress. Honestly, my one position was equal to four of a normal job because of what was expected. I was up to driving 4 hours a day in my territory. Then I took it upon myself to start a new hobby which was my health and wellness business. I started school, which was a one-year program and launched my business, Unwrap You, at the same time in 2013. I had no idea all the responsibility that went along with it at the time. Eager and ready to change the world was all I could think about. Imagine now, my career of managing my multi-million-dollar territory, travel, school, networking, growing a business, and all the other responsibilities. I can now clearly see I had the superwoman mentality, and no idea how it was affecting me.

My body reacted to the stress in a way I never imagined. Fast forward to 2016, keep in mind, I am juggling at least seven major responsibilities in this thing called life. I begin to experience symptoms of fatigue, skin breakouts, not sleeping through the night, and, compulsive behavior related to starting my business. I did not understand why this was going on, so I decided to see my physician. This was confusing because a month before I had a favorable bill of health. Unable to find the root cause of my symptoms, the primary care physician referred me to three different specialists. At this point, I experienced tests that I never knew existed such as bone marrow, cancer and blood screenings. My skin and entire body broke out. I was scared thinking what in the world was happening to my body. The doctors could not find anything with all these test and months going by. Perplexed they continued until I along with another holistic doctor figured it out many months later. I was managing all these responsibilities, and the side effect was my internal body system was off. Plain and simple, I was STRESSED and had no clue. For years, I showed signs but did not recognize them. Finally, my doctor sat me down and "the" talk. She recommended that I leave one of my positions before I killed myself. As I reflect on this story, I have to thank God because I was blessed to finally find out what the problem was after so much time had passed.

The next blessing was my transition into the wellness field and practicing what I shared earlier helped tremendously. I applied the techniques mentioned before which were exercising, prayer/meditation, self-care, and eating properly proved beneficial to me managing the stress. Finally, I chose to leave my 18-year career as a pharma representative and pursue my passion and purpose, which is helping people be proactive with their health not reacting with medicine. Too many times I see people taking pills and having surgery vs changing lifestyles. Not only do I impact females but also the youth whose lives are plagued with responsibilities that can translate to stress. Beware this epidemic is real and can happen to anyone. I'm a living witness! I have experienced the superwoman mentality and thank God I had Unwrap You training and support of family and friends to overcome.

Please take care of yourself this year. Make sure you are investing in yourself and your health. Be selfish this year, make your happiness a priority, and cut out anything that interferes with your well-being. Do not settle for anything less than you deserve.

Stress Facts
- Eight of 10 Americans experience stress
- 75% of office visits are stress-related
- Stress is in the workplace
- Financial worries contribute to stress
- Overthinking can lead to stress
- Stress-related illnesses are increasing

The American Medical Association has noted that stress is the underlying cause of more than 60 percent of all human illnesses and diseases. These statistics are important because they are often related to taking on too much and not having a balance or making time for self.

Unwrap the New You

Need to Reduce Stress? Need to Sleep Better? Need to Lose Weight? Want to be Healthier? Know your BMI? You have read your solution! I have provided first-hand occurrences and understand lifestyle change is easier said than done. It is ok to seek help and gain accountability. This is exactly what I did after struggling with weight issues. Determined to get healthy, I finally had to seek advice. This is the same help I now provide to clients all over the United States. Plans vary based on the assessment and need, but it is an excellent way to jumpstart your success.

Our programs include:

Level 1 "21 Day Shape Up" online course

Level 2 virtual or live group programs

Level 3 for optimal results working directly with me, Coach Melody.

Everybody is beautiful, but if you don't like something, change it. Your goal should be to become the best YOU. Stay in balance, small things can get you off course. There is not a quick fix to lifestyle change, but the journey is ongoing to create the best you. It is important to walk in your purpose by staying determined and focused. You can achieve any goal you set. Make sure you have the right plan and strategy, if you need to pivot along the way, it is ok.

Coach Melody's Tips:

- Drink water to hydrate the body
- Eat smaller portions
- Stay active by doing what you enjoy
- Walk and talk
- Daily Self-care
- Eat to nourish your body
- Connect socially
- Get plenty of sleep
- Make quality time for self

My goal is to educate and improve health outcomes by helping people alter lifestyles and make sustainable changes. What are the top three takeaways you have from this chapter? Take those and build your wellness program in small steps, be kind to yourself, remember it will not happen overnight. Each reader will have a different cause and effect but be authentic and build the outcome best for you. The goal here is to work towards building a sharp mind, body, and soul. Release the superwoman mentality and begin to live your best life. Health is Wealth!

ABOUT THE AUTHOR

Melody McClellan, aka Coach Melody, is the President of Unwrap You LLC, (Health and Wellness) which focuses on nutrition, health, and exercise. She is a published author of two books; Unwrap the New You Interactive Wellness Journal and Ohhmazing Wellness, Your Dreams are Possible. Coach Melody received the 2017 Excellence in Health Care Award and has over 19 years of experience in the health field, specifically in the areas of diabetes, cholesterol, obesity, and weight management.

She creates an implements corporate wellness programs, develops personalized workshops, facilitates lunch, and learns youth wellness/life skills, and is a dynamic speaker. Her goal is to educate and improve health outcomes.

In addition to her passion for health and wellness, Coach Melody is an ambassador for the American Heart Association, and a life member of Alpha Kappa Alpha Sorority, Inc. She has been married for 24 years and has two amazing sons.

Contact Coach Melody at:

- Web: www.unwrapyou.com
- Email: coachmelody@unwrapyou.com
- Instagram: @coachmelody
- Linkedin: @coachmelody
- Facebook: unwrap you with coach melody

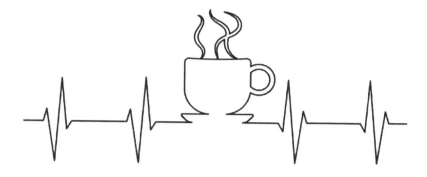

The Courage to Continue

By Dr. Michelle V. Knights

From the beginning of time, the quest for the fountain of youth was fierce. It was one that only the most courageous embarked upon.

It was mythical, mystical, and mysterious...escaping even the most prolific, elite women who sought to reverse the devastation of the aging process and all that it brings with it: disease, decline, and devaluation. Throughout history, a strong emphasis on physical beauty served as an indicator of status, happiness, wealth, and of course, health. After all, health emanates from the inside out, so a woman's appearance seemed reasonable as a measure of living an abundant, quality life. However, lifestyle and dietary practices across the ages didn't promote the fountain of youth. There was an urgency to discover this fountain for women to tap into this elusive wonder. The fountain of youth was highly sought after because women did not understand the transformative power of doing the internal work of adopting sound health principles into daily living. Health is built on the fundamentals of nurturing and nourishing the mind, body, and soul. Our goal is to create the best version of ourselves, one that is stronger, more resilient, more determined, mentally, physically, and spiritually – to live with the courage to continue. It is within our capacity to face our fears with faith because faith gives us courage to believe in ourselves. Fear and faith cannot occupy the same space. Without faith, there can be no courage. Be decisive, have the courage to continue the pursuit for the fountain of youth, when others have lost their way.

As a young girl, I grew up in paradise, a place where the fountain of youth seemed to be everywhere with all the beauty of nature, holistic living and natural remedies practiced daily, empowering women to be healthy and happy. Our island boasts of biodiversity, untouched natural beauty, vibrant culture comprised of a unique blend of people, distinctive heritage, rhythmic calypso, and delectable savory food everywhere. Everyone unreservedly embarks upon the richness of natural living, immerses oneself in the comforts of life, steals away with the sounds of sweet steel pan music, and engages in a laid back "don't worry, be happy" kind of cultural mantra. The majestic twin islands of Trinidad and Tobago (T&T), my paradise, filled with the most precious memories in the making of my youth, certainly empowered me to have the courage to continue my journey. Living in Tobago, I experienced the tranquility of the ocean with white sandy beaches touching the blue skies, being awakened by the robust sounds of roosters with their cock-a-doodle-doo with the hopeful sunrise in the distant horizon. The early morning air always fresh and crisp, was filled with the aroma of every fruit one could ever desire — mangoes, plums, pineapples, guavas and that's just in my backyard. We lived in abundance in a very healthy, natural, holistic environment. We delighted in picking the fresh mangoes from the trees paying no attention to the numerous fallen ones left for the birds and chickens to feast. Everything we consumed came from the earth or animals we raised. We planted cassava, potatoes, corn, avocados, and peanuts, to name a few. With scores of coconut trees around us blooming and laden, we refreshed our bodies from the hot tropical heat with the cooling effects of satisfying coconut water. One of my favorite activities was going fishing with my grandmother and uncles in the bay. We walked a mile to get to the beach and entered the small bay section where we would cast our worn-out well-used nets always catching enough fish to break them. Upon arrival back home, my grandmother gave me bottles filled with milk from our cows to make cheese and butter. Did I mention the savory aroma of freshly homemade bread baked in dirt ovens? It was a cherished weekly ritual, baking delicious and wholesome bread, for the family.

One would think that with such a healthy lifestyle, the discovery of the fountain of youth would be easily achieved – it was quite the contrary. Although this abundance of natural healthy food and lifestyle was the way of life, an interesting phenomenon was happening in the culture and continued to get worse over the next several decades progressively.

People were battling with chronic diseases. Diabetes, hypertension, and heart attacks were among the things that plagued my people. How could this happen in the midst of paradise where everything needed for healthy living was available in abundance? Studies were conducted to assess the prevalence and contributing factors of these emerging widespread health concerns. One major indicator was education. Knowledge about health principles and how to incorporate them in daily living was desperately needed. So, getting back to the basics, where food is used for healing and not just pleasure, is essential. Understanding that mind, body, and soul are interconnected, and what you're eating as well as what's eating you contribute to you achieving lasting health and happiness.

As I left the pristine environment of my island haven and migrated to the U.S.A, I experienced a different type of abundance. My quest continued to find the fountain of youth in America, and while it was everywhere, it seemed invisible to most. American culture, a complex blend of many diverse cultures, reflected a love of food, recreation, leisure, work and going after the American dream. With unlimited food options including fast foods, ethnic, healthy, and comfort foods, there seemed to be a deficit of nutrient-rich foods as a quick and easy option for busy families who were struggling to get by in the middle class. A trend of vegetarian and vegan lifestyles increases, but these seem to be more exclusive rather than inclusive to the general population. Like many Americans, I too fell prey the easy access of food coupled with living a stressful lifestyle. My mind, body, and spirit suffered as a consequence.

Quite interestingly, like Caribbean culture, there is a need for education about health and the power of adapting a principled life to experience health and happiness. In American culture with plenty of food available some only experience limited choices in the food economy and have to relearn everything, they know about food and its connection to diseases and health. There is nothing so empowering as learning and developing the courage to extend your life, and true learning requires unlearning and relearning.

In contrast to the US, people in T&T have lived on more nutrient-dense plant-based foods; however, they have to relearn principles that educate about the real fountain of youth. Unlike the American culture, where many are challenged with eating healthy foods because they grew up on fast foods and TV dinners, high sugar cereals and bagels for breakfast, and now learn how to make healthy choices, this was not the experience of people in my generation or my culture. Yet, the emerging phenomenon of unhealthy outcomes in my paradise is seen everywhere. One indicator of why this might be happening is the lack of education around proper utilization of all the resources around them.

While it's easy to point out the accessibility of fast foods in American culture and prevalence of food insecurity, there is also an overwhelming abundance of healthy options, but like T&T education is needed to help people make comprehensive healthy choices, and this requires the courage to continue the journey.

Without the infrastructures for proper education, people resort to things that media and society ascribe value to, even if they cause more harm than good. So, the quick, easy fixes to become healthy and happy like plastic surgery, bariatric surgery, breast and butt implants, and other interventions often result in further complications, rather than doing the internal work and making sustainable dietary and lifestyle changes. The cost of maintaining youth, health, and wellness is more than mere dollars spent on medical procedures and includes psychological, emotional, and physical costs as well. A closer look at cost of looking younger and healthier reveals cultural influences on what we value from teeth to skin, hair, and weight. Before the popularizing of plastic surgery, to look younger and healthier, women turned to herbs as a natural remedy, albeit extreme at times including crocodiles as an exotic additive. We've come a long way from Victorian women using mercury to get rid of acne and wrinkles, dangerously destroying the skin, to now using placenta and leeches to restore our healthy youthful look, yet somehow the fountain of youth evades us. The essence of good health, radiance, youthfulness, and happiness do not have to be extreme or elusive. In fact, it is accessible, attainable, and available to everyone regardless of age, social class, culture, or geography, but it requires a commitment to courage.

Some constants determine great health outcomes, and these revolve around eight natural laws of health that govern our lives and give us the courage to continue implementing these when we want to give up. These principles enable us to live optimally resilient and fulfilled lives, but often they are ignored, grossly trampled upon and destroyed. These natural laws are the fountain of youth. They are supported by science and research and transcend cultural nuances. They are not arduous but are powerfully profound yet simple; creating and stimulating a universal culture of empowering women to increase wellness, health, and happiness.

Health is a language everyone speaks, and these foundational principles can be remembered with the acronym **START NOW**.

Principle #1 – Sunlight

One of nature's most healing remedies, it is powerful for physical, emotional, and mental health and wellbeing, and Vitamin D deficiencies. It provides the basis for all life.

Principle #2 – Temperance

We have all heard the saying, "be moderate or temperate in all things." This includes every aspect of our lives, including what we eat and drink. This means balancing our responsibilities of caregiving, nurturing, and self-care. Refresh and recharge so you can show up stronger and healthier for yourself and your family.

Principle #3 – Activity

The power of activity through exercise cannot be overstated. Science has indicated women should exercise 3-4 times per week to reduce high blood pressure, reduce stress, boost endurance, and strengthen mind and body. Exercise releases feel-good, and happiness hormones that increases blood flow and proper circulation gets more oxygen to the brain, muscles, and organs so you can meet all the multiple demands of your life.

Principle #4 – **R**est

The power of rest is often overlooked in our society. Sleep deprivation is one of the causes of accidents and many health problems. Even a short power nap can improve productivity and alertness, lowers heart disease, and stress-related illnesses.

Rest and relaxation lead to mental clarity, creativity, and deeper, thoughtful decisions.

Principle #5 – **T**rust in Divine Power

This is an important principle because it connects us to the true healer. It is pivotal, a spiritual dimension that provides supernatural power and peace to facilitate and fulfill all the other laws. Stress and worry are counterproductive to good health and happiness; they wear out the life forces resulting in increased health issues, disease, and eventual death. Conversely, faith, and trust in a higher power, surrendering, and submitting in obedience leads to relinquishing burdens and finding peace and happiness that surpasses understanding.

Additionally, studies indicate that the power of belief, confidence, and prayer to God contributes to health and healing. Research also indicates a link between beliefs and wellbeing, i.e., life satisfaction, hope, purpose, and meaning, are linked to lower rates of depression, less anxiety, less anger, lower suicide rates, more optimism, and hope.

Furthermore, women live a life of gratitude and benevolence when they trust in God.

Principle #6 – **Nutrition**

We are what we eat, and we have a responsibility to nourish our bodies. Proper nutrition enables us to face and break cultural, cultivated and emotional eating habits, and addresses when and what you eat, as well as discouraging eating between meals. Reducing or eliminating sugars in your diet is critical to health mastery.

Sugar is the world's third most commercially valuable crop yet yields no benefit to humanity. Instead, it produces a global epidemic of a wide range of health crises. Obesity and related diseases such as dementia, cancer, diabetes, and heart disease are present wherever sugar-based foods dominate the lifestyle. While sugar needs to be diminished, it's important to limit fat intake as that is more dangerous to triggering diabetes than sugar.

Principle #7 – **O**xygen

Pure air filling the lungs providing adequate supplies of oxygen to the body allows for improved health and functioning. Exposure to toxins and polluted air compromises functioning of organs and leads to greater susceptibility of diseases. Polluted air in and out of the home environment contributes to the onset or exacerbation of lung cancer, respiratory diseases, brain and nerve damage, and heart disease.

Principle #8 – **W**ater

Water intake is critical and is synonymous with life itself; it contains elements of life and sustains it. We are made up of 75% water, and every cell needs to be hydrated. Drink at least 6-8 cups of water each day. Many people live a very dehydrated life, which contributes to health issues. Every process in our bodies depends on water for their optimal functioning. The root of many problems lies with inadequate water intake. Profoundly, water consumption can even stop preterm labor. Without water, life would cease to exist.

While each component is powerful, the whole of these eight health principles are greater than the sum of its parts, thanks to its synergistic effects. Incorporating these simple principles of health will give you the strongest foundation for building a healthier, happier more fulfilled you, and extend the youthfulness and vibrancy of your life. Adapting these eight health principles will be fueled by what you value most in life.

This brings us to a pivotal point of focusing on values, the fountain of transformation. What we value gets held in high esteem of importance and worth, allowing us to create the future we want. Further, what we value gets our attention and resources. To be guided by our values requires an embracing of a principled life. Dr. Spencer Holman developed a philosophy based on 10 Life Values, which purports that to live a life of value, one must do the internal work of examining one's life.

His work addresses the famous dictum of ancient philosophers who stated that "an unexamined life is not worth living," and he designed the construct scaffolding the principle that living on the foundation of the 10 Life Values creates a conduit to fulfillment and excellence. His philosophy outlines the role of values and systems to orchestrate an effective process for examining every aspect of an ordered and principled life. The 10 Life Values are an inclusive collection, an interrelated system which encompasses a unified approach focusing on values of:

Spiritual, Health, Family, Appearance, Dwelling, Mobility, Education, Profession, Leisure and Wealth, all of which promote reflection and a new paradigm for achieving an examined life, regardless of cultural influences.

It establishes accountability as the cornerstone of success. Living an unexamined life has serious and lasting implications, but collaboratively, we demonstrate the courage to continue and create opportunities to manifest the discovery of the true internal fountain of youth. One such effort led to our creation of The Society of Womanhood Elevation (WE), where we move women from stagnation to significance using the principles of the 10 Life Values to empower and support women in achieving powerful, healthy and happy lives. This requires discipline for achieving the principled life. My health journey has been empowered by using these principles contained within the health value system. I am healthier and stronger having achieved my weight loss goals and increased my vitality and overall sense of wellbeing. Consequently, I am more fulfilled having experienced bliss, health, and happiness.

Winston Churchill said, "Success is not final; failure is not fatal; it is the courage to continue that counts." The path of your journey towards health can be difficult or overwhelming; particularly without a system that offers you the blueprint to success. It will take organizing your life, having a sequential, progressive plan that you can grow into and is responsive to the needs of your life and your family. Most of all, it will require courage to continue when you've plateaued, or you're not producing favorable results.

Remember that you didn't develop unhealthy habits and patterns overnight; therefore, reversing these behaviors will take time. Be patient with yourself – believe that everything you need is accessible to you, start there; keep educating yourself, and take action. Be bold; we don't need more degrees, more experience, and more time, what we need is more courage to believe now. Embrace all your experiences for they have made you who you are today, go to your core, celebrate yourself, and transform your life with manageable changes. It's time to go back to the basics; there you will find life more abundantly. Live life with more courage to step out and go against conventional thinking and the norms we accept as truth. Have the courage to question our assumptions about surviving in a hectic society, more courage to get into action not knowing what lies ahead, but believing we are worthy of the amazing energized life that's waiting on the other side of fear if only we dare to believe and act.

Develop the courage to continue your health journey understanding the interlocking nature of your mind, body and soul, and the courage to continue on the path to an examined life, one worth living on the foundation of 10 Life Values. When we're young we have youth, as we get older we want youth to return, but if we carry this fountain of youth with us on our journey, as a source of infinite goodness rather than a place or destination, then we would always be inspired to have the courage to continue our pursuit of health and happiness. **S**unlight, **T**emperance, **A**ctivity, **R**est, **T**rust in Divine Power, **N**utrition, **O**xygen, and **W**ater – remember, every woman dares to continue because you carry your fountain of YOUTH with you everywhere you go so START NOW!

ABOUT THE AUTHOR

Dr. Michelle V. Knights is an innovative thought leader, professor, strategist, transformational and peak performance coach, author, and international speaker. Her work has impacted individuals and communities around the world. She has a Ph.D. in Human Development and Family Studies and has served as faculty at University of Prince Edward Island, Canada; Messiah College, and Penn State University in the US. She has worked with international entities, state government, and local organizations to stimulate transformation, productivity, and growth. She focuses on enriching lives through the examination of values to create intergenerational and multigenerational empowerment and success.

Dr. Michelle has helped companies and individuals expand their growth in a corporate environment, as entrepreneurs, and as subject matter experts and has developed individuals to leadership status and top producers. She has experienced business successes such as facilitating business growth and strategy development, trained and coached leaders and their teams in sales, mindset, and personal development, and consulted with companies to improve development strategy. Dr. Michelle serves as the Business Development Director for AGame, improving the lives of men, and has helped the company increase international exposure. Currently, Dr. Michelle has launched a platform for transformational peak performance success called The Society of Womanhood Elevation, WE, helping move women from stagnation to significance. She is dedicated to serving all who are in quest of a fulfilled examined life. She understands the importance of reinventing oneself, nurturing a family, combining passion, purpose, and power to be unstoppable, and believes that all things are possible.

To contact Dr. Michelle Knights please call (302) 897-9690 or email DrMichelleKnights@gmail.com

To learn more about AGame visit
https://agameformen.com

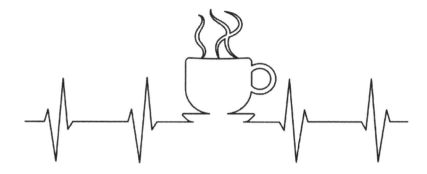

Your Livelihood is Killing You
By Radiah Rhodes, CPC

I am a fan of routines. I had always thought of routines as a way to help us get things done efficiently while at the same time, giving us a sense of control and security. I believe this is the case for healthy routines, where you're aware of the purpose and elements of the routine and how they help you achieve your goals. However, on the flip side, routines are very similar to practice. You get out what you put in. I learned the hard way that all routines are not good routines. They are generic structures that can produce positive and healthy outcomes just as easily as they can produce negative outcomes that diminish your health. It all depends on the actions that make up the routine and how conscious, aware, and intentional you are about the routine you're following.

I used to be masterful at holding it all together. As a wife, mother, executive, and a Black Woman, I could keep it moving, make it happen, figure it out, and look good while doing it. I had a mountain of competing responsibilities, and just like every working mother I knew, I constantly wished for more time, energy, and money to get it all done. I had the standard agenda of work activities, travel, and deadlines, kids school programs, and sports schedules, social events with family and friends, and maybe some "me" time tucked in there somewhere. It was an isolated moment to rest and feel at peace when I had to handle everything life was demanding. Not only was I physically and mentally exhausted, but the constant grind also drained my soul.

Every couple of months, I battled chronic sinus infections, which turned into the cough that never goes away. The congestion by itself was enough to drive me crazy. When you can't breathe, everything is compromised. Sleep was minimal, exercise was non-existent, and my energy was at an all-time low. Mentally, I was constantly on edge and ready to snap at the smallest things.

6:30 am

Mornings were the worst. Waking up after a restless night of semi-sleep and getting myself dressed while getting two elementary school children up and out to school was a daily trauma. The school day didn't start until 9:23 am, but we were all awake by 6:30 am. If I stayed focused, I could get a work out in. Otherwise, the morning routine dragged out and overlapped with the first meetings of the day. That was a sure recipe for chaos. The mute button cannot save you from a child determined to get your attention. By the time I got in the car for my forty-five-minute commute, I had wished the day was over, and it had barely gotten started.

9:00 am

Traffic. The best-case scenario was a forty-five-minute "highway hypnotized" ride through clear weather with no accidents. My commute had never been an issue before, but once I hit the limit of exhaustion, it was a wrap. It was a struggle to stay awake and focus on the road. I moved to a flexible work arrangement to manage the commute. I worked from home two days a week as a way to work out the situation and keep going. I regularly scheduled conference calls on the days I had to drive, but I still zoned out. It was like muscle memory; I was stuck in a pattern that kicked in as soon as I hit the highway. It wore me down, but I just kept it moving.

10:00am

Once I got to the office, I'd have to sit at my desk for a good fifteen minutes to get it together and get some energy flowing. It would feel like it was 10 pm, but the clock only read 10 am, so I still had the full workday in front of me. This might not have been so bad if I was excited about my job, but nope, that was not the case. The day job saga is a whole book in itself, but let me give you the top three highlights. First, I was in my sixteenth year at the company after deciding way back in year one, that I wanted to leave. Who does that?! Second, after all of these years, I was finally bringing "my authentic self" to work, and that made me a problem. Third, the environment had become as toxic as I had become authentic, and the conflict made me sick. Remember those sinus infections? This was not a random coincidence. The stress of my workday was compromising my immune system and keeping me in a cycle of sickness I couldn't shake. Month after month my doctor would tell me, you have to stop. That wasn't an option in my world. I had to work. This was my livelihood. This is who I was, and it was essential to my identity. I worked hard, I put in the effort, and I held it together. Leaving my job was not a decision I was willing to make.

5:00pm

The Healthy Hour. Every Monday, Tuesday, and Wednesday, I had an appointment scheduled like clockwork. I faithfully checked in at 5 pm at an upscale health and vitality center for my self-care. On Monday was acupuncture, Tuesday's was massage, and on Wednesday's I had a vitamin IV flush. For thirty to sixty minutes, I sat quiet, still, and relaxed. I closed my eyes, breathed deeply, and enjoyed every minute of my treatment. I walked out refreshed and ready for the next phase of the day.

6:00pm

The "Six O'Clock Scramble" begins. Sports practice, homework, dinner, baths, and bedtime…for the children, not for me. The third commute of the day, my husband and I would divide and conquer. We'd each navigate rush hour traffic through town, to pick up each child and get them to practices. This was a blur of changing clothes and finding equipment, water bottles, and cleats so we could get out of the door and back on the road. Practice time was precious.

The children were safe and occupied. I had a full uninterrupted ninety-minute stretch to get back to work. Hotspot, laptop, and phone in hand, it was like I'd never left the office.

The effects of my "Healthy Hour" were over and done with. It became clear that my self-care routine was actually glammed up life support. Although I had some powerful practices, they were no match for my schedule. My Monday, Tuesday, Wednesday regimen was barely helping me survive the load of my work and lifestyle.

8:30 pm

The night shift. Once we all got home, it was time for homework and dinner. There was a 50/50 chance that homework would go smoothly and a 50/50 chance we were eating a home-cooked meal vs. takeout. Both homework and dinner had a significant impact on how the night ended. On a good night, we had independent self-study and a healthy-ish meal that could be prepared in less than thirty minutes. This meant we could all be asleep or relaxing by about 9:30 pm and I could wind down without feeling frazzled by common core or having indigestion from takeout. On the rough nights, it went down completely different. There was confusion over the assignments, a frustration with every problem, and zero patience to work through the struggle. Multiply that times, two children and add to it a pizza or something heavy and unhealthy for dinner, and the night became brutal. Tears, stomach aches, falling asleep at the table, lectures on focus, Google, Siri, Alexa…everybody was tired and worn out.

10:00pm

Time to log back in and pick up where I left off during practice. Another email check, finishing up a few notes and documents, glancing at tomorrow's schedule and maybe even prepping for the day's meetings. By this time, I was delirious and the only reason I didn't feel guilty for being glued to my laptop is because my husband was glued to his too. Some nights I'd try to shut down my computer and read a little before I went to sleep. I lasted about two pages and usually woke up with the book still in my hands or lightly resting on my face. I'd look over, and my husband was asleep. Still dressed in his clothes from the day. Why were we choosing to live like this?

12:00 am

Sleep. Until about 3:00 am or 3:30 am when my brain would start buzzing, and I'd have to grab a pen and paper to document all of the thoughts running through my mind. Then I'd lay back down until 6:30 am, wake up and do it all over again.

Wake up. Work it. Burn Out. Repeat.

This was my daily routine. Day in and day out, I would get up, get it together, make it happen, and figure out how to reach the finish line at the end of each day. This was my own personal, yet all too common, pattern of insanity. I am not unique. This is the textbook lifestyle of many working women and mothers around the globe.

And although it is easy to rationalize that we should be grateful because so many people in the world deal with more serious issues, this issue remains a toxic reality that is leading women directly to burnout and illness. That is serious enough for me.

I couldn't see the forest for the trees in my madness. I was on autopilot, stuck in a default pattern trying to survive. I'm not even sure if I would've stopped if I hadn't gotten sick. Finally, it was the truth that I could no longer deny or resist. I had driven myself to chronic illness, and I had to stop before it got worse. My doctor put me on medical leave, and I took time off to heal and get well. It was the equivalent of a signed permission slip to save myself. Over the next few days, I became lucid and resolved. I went to work to deliver the message that I'd be out for a few weeks, but my soul knew it was my last day. I was emotional and relieved all at the same time. I could finally let go and allow myself to rest.

My job was my livelihood. Over time, I had unconsciously made it the anchor of my identity, esteem, and security. Even though I was financially stable and I had other hobbies and pursuits; I had mentally and emotionally made the paycheck, benefits, and perks from that one job the sole source of my identity and survival. It was a severe blind spot. I'm a certified coach, a master energy practitioner, and a designer of self-actualization products, but I could not get out of my way when it came to my livelihood. It was the last frontier, and once I was released, I committed to going all-in on living well and being free.

In hindsight, my journey was simple. I had a trigger incident with my health that woke me up. I finally chose to listen, and then I moved through three phases to recover, restore, and renew.

SHIFT-IT

I had to stop with the "self-care" conversation and call "a thing, a thing." I was out there calling grooming, travel, and damage repair, self-care. That perspective kept me believing that a bunch of activities, departure dates, and appointments were enough to keep me whole and well. Yes, vacations and massages were ways to care for my body, but they did not get to the source of what was breaking me down. They were great ways to escape and put a band-aid on what was causing the issues for the moment, but I still had to go back to the same pattern.

I was too afraid to go deep and uncover the root of what was driving my stress. It scared me to think that I might have to leave my job, and if I did, I knew my husband would not have agreed with me. Every time I would go down that path, I would start catastrophizing the situation. I'd go from A to Z in two seconds. I'd start with saying to myself, "Radiah, tell the truth." And the next thing you know, I'd be thinking

I had to leave it all, become a Yogi, and "Eat, Pray, Love" my way to a better life. So I would just cut off the process and refuse to go deep down to my truth. It was easier to escape it with a quick trip, a new outfit, or the latest motivational book.

I had to shift out of this whole mode of thinking and living. Thinking I had to ruin my entire life to make the important choices were keeping paralyzed. I stayed on a roller coaster of living between struggling, sacrificing, and settling for a life that was good enough.

I had a great family, a good job, and the luxury perks, but I didn't have peace, satisfaction, nor fulfillment. Being highly educated, experienced, and accomplished didn't make me as happy as I'd hoped it would. The "good life" trappings became the trap that was, not only keeping me from reaching great goals, impact, and real fulfillment; it was keeping me from a basic level of health and wellness.

Confronting the reality and risk of my declining health was the trigger. I don't recommend letting it go that far when you can heed the early signs. You know if you're stressed more than is healthy for you. You know if you're having physical symptoms of exhaustion, anxiety, or even digestive issues. If you don't, start with taking the time to get to know yourself and your body. Ask yourself questions like "Is this how I want to feel?" or " how is this situation working for me?" If you ask in earnest, you will get a clear answer. Honor the clear solution, even if it's just writing and speaking a declaration of your truth. "This situation is not working for me, and I am committed to shifting it." Start there, tell your truth and then embrace it and share it with someone you trust to support and hold you accountable to it. That's the shift, from avoiding and denying your truth to acknowledging and speaking it out loud. It takes the willingness to make one powerful declaration and then honor it one step at a time.

OWN IT

Now that you know your truth, you can own it. Ownership is power. When you own something, you can expand and leverage it for greater returns. So many times, we think taking ownership is a burden or that it requires too much responsibility. It requires trust, but you are already completely "able to respond" to whatever situations come up. You're already doing it; you might as well do it under the circumstances you desire and enjoy.

The bottom line is, you take care of what you own. You invest in what you own. You develop and grow what you own. Own your truth, own your power, and own your well-being by making choices that feed your health and free you up. What choices do you need to make to free up your time, energy, and money? Take inventory and write down what's taking up your resources. Do a quick audit of everywhere you spend time, energy, and money and choose to either continue or stop engaging every item on the list. You might decide to continue the same activities but do so knowing you're making a conscious choice. You do not have to become a victim of your fear. Everyone's circumstances are different, and there might be one million valid reasons to "not make a choice," but that is still choosing.

There will always be reasons, and they will seem very, very real. The gravity of those reasons will be enough to keep you in the same orbit…the same orbit that's getting you what you've got. You will always be able to rationalize and justify staying in the same pattern and I would bet money that you will be "just fine." If "just fine" is the truth and it works, then read no further. But if it doesn't, you will have to get good at choosing.

Be willing to choose what serves you over what drains your most valuable resources…because you say so. You don't need a reason for it, you don't need to earn it, and you don't need to convince anyone about your choice. It's yours, own it. Then, be strategic and deliberate about focusing your energy on what you're choosing and creating. The other items will take care of themselves, and if there is anything for you to do about them, you'll know and be able to respond.

Remember when you own something, you care for it, you invest in it, and you leverage it. What are you owning? Owners are confident, strategic, decisive, committed, etc. Choose what works and then become an owner in how you manage it.

LIVE IT

As far as we know, this is our one life. Exist in it or live it, it's up to you. I'm going to keep this simple. Once you shift from denial to truth, and once you own your power, align everything in your life around that truth and power. Period.

Look at your schedule, your connections, your work, your home space, your refrigerator, and everything else. Look at all of it and choose only what aligns with your truth. The focus is on YOU, not what's falling away or fighting you to stay. It's on you, what you're building, and how you're choosing to live. These are the greater returns. First you **SHIFT-IT**, then you **OWN IT**, and finally, you **LIVE IT**. Every day, wake up, work it, wind down, and repeat only the things that serve your truth and power.

ABOUT THE AUTHOR

Author Radiah Rhodes is passionate about power. As a well-being activist, energy practitioner, and twenty-year veteran of Fortune 100 corporate America, she has mastered the spirit, science, and reality of authentic power and trains hundreds of people each year on how to access and leverage their innate power to succeed.

www.evoklife.com
info@evoklife.com
IG @evoklife @radiahrhodes

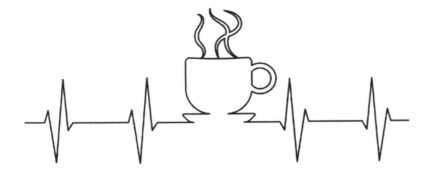

How to Have A Great Day
By Stacey Brass-Russell

There are very few things, or so it seems, in this world that are truly in our control. We go through life doing our very best to navigate the twists and turns that unexpectedly show up on our path as well as the thoughts and emotions that accompany them. It's a roller-coaster at best, and we are the riders, experiencing the highs, lows, and everything in between.

Many of us start to play "defense" in the game of life and get into habits and routines that become all about how to "get through" the day while barely getting by. Time seems to shapeshift – we have less of it when we want more and more of it when we want less. We wonder why it's so difficult to have what we would like – more ease, more peace, less stress, and no conflict. And so we live at a deficit. There's never enough sleep, so we press snooze until the last minute and then rush to get to our first activity of the day. We eat on the run, picking up convenient food that seems like it will satisfy our needs. When, in fact, it lacks the nourishment required to truly feed our bodies and create the energy we need. We drag. We plan to do things that are important for our well-being "later" and then the day gets away from us leaving those good intentions for exercise, relaxation or making a home-cooked meal left behind. But maybe the biggest challenge of all is managing our thoughts. Constantly on sensory overload we are inundated with news, social media, images and experiences that leave us raw, reactive and ready for a fight.

Does any of this sound familiar to you? It's a description of "being out of alignment." Simply put, this is when you have not established a foundation of health and well-being for yourself that connects you to the inherent rhythm of nature and the universe before exposing yourself to all of the external influences that you face each day. Your alignment is made up essentially of two things – what I call your "inner game" and your "outer game." Your inner game is your mindset, emotional well-being, your sense of self, and feeling of connection. Your "outer game" is your actions and choices that you make daily, including how you interact with others, how you take care of your physical body and the activities you engage in.

The great news is that with a few simple adjustments, you can learn how to align your inner and outer game and start living in the flow of things. A few years ago, I made some shifts that changed how I was living in alignment, and I now teach this to my clients. It's all about knowing what *IS* in your control and maximizing that to your advantage before you get into the part of your day that is largely *NOT* in your control and having better tools for managing and handling that reality.

When I was ten years old, I was in the original Broadway production of ANNIE. While this was one of the most positive and incredible experiences of my life, it also informed a lot of my "identity" and habits that I carried with me well into adulthood. I used to get home from the theatre around 11:30 pm still full of energy. I would have a snack, watch TV, sleep in and then arrive at school late to accommodate my 8 shows a week schedule. Over these two years I adopted the "night owl" lifestyle of show business.

When I was 33 years old, I completed my first yoga teacher training certification and started teaching. I had been practicing yoga and making conscious changes to my lifestyle – exploring different nutrition and wellness recommendations and slowly shifting into a healthier version of myself. Over the next 15 years, I became more knowledgeable and more aligned in most ways – except one. I had never undone the "night owl" habits that had been in place since I was ten years old. It wasn't until a friend invited me to join a group health coaching program focused on healthy habits that I even considered that this way of operating could be outdated for me. During this ten-week program we re-examined our rituals and routines and for me, what emerged was a new understanding of how my morning could make or break the entire rest of my day.

That spring, I enrolled in a program to become a health and life coach and ended up becoming a master level, transformational coach. As a coach I started to see how all of my knowledge and passion about yoga, breathing, meditation, nutrition, energy, the nervous system and connection to the Universe could come together to create a morning system that addressed this major issue that we face as humans every day – how to get into and stay in alignment. From the moment we step outside our doors, we are subjected to external influences completely out of our control. Our senses are accosted, our internal rhythm and relationship to time get high-jacked, and our nervous system starts processing information and making meaning of our experiences. Many of us indeed have families to interact with before we ever even encounter the outside world, but even so we each need to figure out how to carve out the time to take care of ourselves before we can take care of others. How can we maintain physical, emotional, and spiritual balance as we go about our days? How can we create inner strength and stability for ourselves so that we may respond to the needs of our lives with clarity, grace and an open heart? In answering this question for myself, I created a system that I call "How to Have A Great Day." We can never have any way of knowing what each day will bring, but we can do our very best to set ourselves up for success.

Here is my fool-proof formula for getting yourself ready to face the day with inner and outer alignment and a general sense of health and well-being:

1. **<u>Wake Up Early</u>**

   Cultivating this habit was a game-changer for me. As an experiment, I started pushing my wake-up time back a little earlier until I found the ideal amount of time that I enjoyed having in the morning before my first appointment or obligation. Because I did it gradually, it didn't feel hard.

   Waking up early is the only way to ensure that you can have space and time to do the things that you know are important for your self-care. This may mean having ample time to enjoy the inherent expansiveness that comes with the morning hours. As you become more tuned in, you will notice that the energy of the morning is very different than that of the afternoon or evening. It is considered to be a time of creativity often referred to as "the time of the Gods" and most beneficial for the quiet practices of meditation and contemplation.

   When you are rushing, your nervous system perceives that as stress and you start producing certain chemicals and hormones that put you into "fight or flight" mode which triggers a whole systemic response that interferes with digestion, circulation, clarity, and expression. Your body has to work harder and therefore, less efficient.

Slowing down is one of the key ingredients to lowering our stress levels and improving our health. The tempo of your day is established in the morning, so making a conscious effort to give yourself more time is a great place to start. This also is the first step in being able to integrate the next four items for having a great day.

2. **Hydrate**

Up until two years ago, the first thing I would put into my stomach upon waking up was coffee. There was even a time that I had an automatic coffee maker with a timer that would start brewing before my alarm went off!

I always knew that drinking water was essential for health, but when I learned that it was important to make water the very first thing that you put into your body each day I changed my habit to water first, coffee second. When you wake up, you are dehydrated. Your body has been fasting for hours and has also been digesting, assimilating, absorbing and getting ready for elimination. Your intestines and colon need water to function (one of the number one causes of constipation is dehydration). To start your metabolism and digestion going you must hydrate and signal your body to wake up. Think of this as "all systems go."

To make this a habit, I started preparing my water the night before. Every night I make my morning water jar which consists of filling a 32 oz — Mason jar with filtered water, freshly squeezed lemon, and slices of cucumber. I leave my jar on my nightstand and the first thing I do in the morning is drink my water. I no longer turn on the TV and drink coffee first. Now I sit quietly, hydrate and breathe (usually with a cat on my lap). This routine has had such a positive impact on how I feel that I literally can't imagine my day without it!

3. **Move a Little**

I used to think that if I didn't have time for a full workout or yoga class that it didn't count. What I wasn't remembering was the simplicity of the fact that our bodies need movement to function. Our spines need to twist and bend to remain lubricated. Our lungs need our rib cages and abdominal muscles to be supple and moveable to expand and contract.

In addition, our emotions and instincts are FELT senses that we need to be connected to. I call this being "embodied."

Our bodies are the miraculous vehicles that we experience life through. Movement is how we connect our emotional intelligence with our physical intelligence so that we can feel sensations, be in tune with ourselves and know when we need to adjust.

Starting your day with 5-10 minutes of stretching, intentional breathing or a yoga pose is the way to ensure that you have circulation, oxygen, and awareness which are three essential ingredients for a healthy body and mind!

4. <u>Manage your Mind</u>

I mentioned earlier that when I started my water habit, I also changed another habit. For years I loved turning on the TV first thing in the morning and watching my favorite local news anchor. I felt like it was an essential part of my day, and I enjoyed it! But what I hadn't considered was the impact this was having on my mind and my nervous system.

When we wake up, our minds are quiet(er) and receptive. We have an opportunity to establish what I call the "lens" through which we would like to view our day. If we immediately turn on outside news and stimuli, we are skipping over this and jumping to having our senses receiving and processing outside information before we have tuned in to our thoughts and feelings.

Cleaning your lens and grounding into space from which you would like to move into the day can be done in any number of ways. Here is a list of some of my favorite ways to manage your mind for the day:

- Meditate
- Journal
- Make a gratitude list
- Handwrite your schedule
- Visualize yourself going through your day with ease
- Pull from a deck of Oracle or Affirmation Cards
- Read or listen to something inspiring

You can do something different every day! I promise that you will be amazed at how adding a 5-minute mindfulness practice into your morning will impact how you show up and interact with others in an extremely positive way.

5. **Nourish**

I used to think that it was fine to have coffee in the morning and then wait hours before eating solid food. I often tricked myself into thinking I wasn't hungry, used it as a weight-loss tool, or didn't give it much thought. I would also often grab something on the go and eat while walking.

Having a proper breakfast at home is one of the best healthy habits you can cultivate. To feel satisfied, have energy and absorb nutrients it is recommended that you have protein, fat, and fiber at every meal and that you eat while relaxed. This means that "who you are being" while you eat is just as important as what you eat when it comes to your metabolism.

My favorite breakfast recommendation for my clients is to make a smoothie that gives you everything you need. My breakfast smoothie has ¼ cup berries, ½ banana, almond butter, baby spinach, oat milk, cinnamon, turmeric, flax seeds, and hemp seeds. It's full of protein, antioxidants, anti-inflammatories, nutrients and fat! Everything to keep me satisfied and energized until lunch.

And that is my system that I call "How to Have a Great Day" – wake up early, hydrate, move your body, manage your mind and nourish. While none of this information is new or groundbreaking, it is the total of doing all 5 of these things every morning that is my secret to success. The beauty in this simple and effective approach to alignment is that every individual can make it their own. What time you wake up is less important than having the time you need to set yourself up for success. How you move your body is totally up to you –do it. Find out what works best for your mindset as long as you have a way to tap into your confidence, power, and positivity every day. And finally, love your body by feeding it nourishing and high-quality foods that you prepare yourself whenever possible. Slow down. Enjoy yourself. Eat when you are relaxed.

On a final note, the human mind tends to compress itself around difficulty and suffering, so it takes some effort to shift things around until we can see the beauty around us. There's work to do to have an open heart and to know that LOVE is your birthright. So do the work – it's worth it. And then go out and have a great day!

ABOUT THE AUTHOR

Stacey Brass-Russell is a Transformational Coach, Yoga Educator & Speaker. She helps creative, purpose-driven individuals do the work they love. Her areas of expertise include organized thinking and action, transforming the mindset and spiritual well-being. Stacey received her Mastery, Health & Life Coaching Certifications from Health Coach Institute and coaches clients all over the world. In addition to attending NYU's Tisch School of the Arts for theatre, Stacey also holds the highest-level yoga teaching certifications available. She resides in New York City with her psychoanalyst husband Christopher and two cats, Ella and Charmaine. She is a passionate home cook, an avid theatre-goer and music lover.

Business: Stacey Brass-Russell Wellness

Website: www.staceybrassrussell.com

Email: stacey@staceybrassrussell.com

FB: https://www.facebook.com/staceybrassrussell/

Instagram:
https://www.instagram.com/staceybrassrussell/?hl=en

Pinterest: https://www.pinterest.com/staceylynnbrass/

LinkedIn: https://www.linkedin.com/in/stacey-brass-russell-1b4921163/

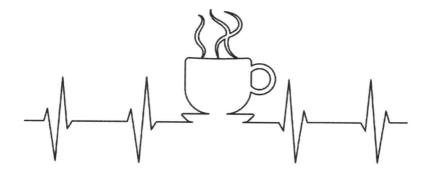

The 15-Day Restorative Detox

By Jeanette Chandler
Dietician and Master of Nutrition

We live in a toxic world. From the moment we wake up in the morning until the time we lay our head back on our pillow, we are under attack. We are exposed to thousands of toxins every single day. Our bodies ingest toxins in the air we breathe, the food we eat, the negative thoughts we play on repeat, and even in the clothes we wear. The scary part is, toxins can wreak havoc on the body in intrusive and long-lasting ways.

To make matters worse, many of us take our bodies for granted. We develop a mindset of overindulgence and misuse, believing our bodies will not suffer the consequences. Rarely do we listen to the internal whispers giving us a heads up when something is off. We push the envelope until our body's ability to naturally remove toxins becomes overwhelmed and can no longer protect us.

The liver plays a vital role in this protection process. When it gets overloaded this is a perfect storm to invite toxins into the bloodstream causing damage to the other systems in our body. As a desperate attempt to grab your attention, a toxic liver will sound the alarm. This alarm is often manifested by the development of troubling conditions such as acne, chronic headaches, psoriasis, inflammatory and autoimmune diseases, and chronic fatigue.

So how do you know if your body needs a tune-up? Ask yourself the following questions and if you answer yes to any of them, it's a clear indication that you may need of a reset.

- Do you often wish you were as vibrant and healthy as other people your age?
- Do you feel sluggish, tired and low energy most days?

- Do you have muscle aches and pains for no apparent reason?
- Is your skin dull, dry or do you have adult acne?

How to choose a detox program?

1. **Consider the reasons why you want to detox** (i.e. better sleep, emotional stability, clearer skin or weight release) Examining your personal reasons can help you pinpoint an ideal detox program. Knowing your "why" will help you stay focused on the road to a healthier happier you! So, what's your why?

2. **Consider the structure of the detox program** (flexible vs. very restrictive)

There is no shortage of theories on the best ways you can reset and restore your body with a detox. Programs range from flexible to extremely restrictive. It's important for you to understand your personality and then choose a detox that aligns with who you are and which program you're most likely to embrace.

3. **Are you ready to change your eating habits?**

Before you begin any detox program there's one very important question you must ask yourself, "Am I ready to change my mindset and habits around food?" Going through a detox program is like hitting the reset button. But if you aren't committed to the idea of embarking on a journey toward a healthier lifestyle, that reset button will have to be pushed over and over again.

4. Consider the duration of the detox program

Detox programs require commitment and takes willpower. The questions you should ask are, how long can I do this? What's my sweet spot? Personally, I find that a 15-day program is not too long, and not too short. Like Goldilocks. It's just right!

5. Evaluate safety

When considering a detox program, safety should always be your priority. The process of removing toxins from your body may cause some withdrawal like effects so it is vital to choose a program that is designed to detox your body safely.

Now, let's get this detox party started!

15 Day Detox Food and Grocery List

Vegetables
Onions, garlic, beets, artichokes, green beans, bok choy and cruciferous vegetables like broccoli, cauliflower, cabbage,

collard greens, kale, and Brussel sprouts.

Other vegetables to eat include asparagus, bell peppers, carrots, celery, cucumbers, endives, jicama, kohlrabi, leeks, lettuce, okra, parsnips, radishes, rutabaga, snow peas, tomatoes, spinach, sprouts, squash, sweet potatoes, turnips, watercress, yams, yucca, and zucchini.

Fruits Whole And Organic
apples, apricots, blackberries, blueberries, cantaloupe, cherries, cranberries, grapefruit, figs, grapes, guava, kiwi, lemon, lime, loganberries, mango, melon, nectarines, oranges, papaya, peaches, pears, pineapple, plums, pomegranate, prunes, raspberries, strawberries, tangerines, and watermelon.

Natural Whole Grains Gluten Free
Amaranth, buckwheat, millet, quinoa, brown rice

Beans and Legumes
Split yellow and green peas.
Lentils (red, brown, green, yellow, French. Other beans and legumes, such as adzuki, cannellini, chickpeas, black, black-eyed peas, kidney, and lima.

Fats
Avocado
butter
Almonds
Brazil nut
Cashew
Chia
Hazelnut
Hemp seeds, hemp nuts, hemp hearts
Macadamia Nut
Pecan

Pine nut
Pistachio
Pumpkin
Sesame seeds
Sunflower seeds
Flax seeds
Poppy Seeds
Walnuts
Coconut

Oils Organic high quality unrefined
Olive
Walnut
Coconut
Sesame
Safflower
Flax tofu

Condiments
Red, Balsamic and Rice Vinegar
Sea Salt, fresh herbs, black pepper, cayenne pepper
Lemons and Limes to taste as salad dressing.
Olives
Tofu

Day 1

Morning detox water: 1 full cup (8 oz) of warm water
with ½ of a lemon

Morning meditation and deep breathing:
What are your intentions for today?

What will you appreciate yourself for today?

What is your water intake goal for today?

Breakfast: Vegetable Juice
½ Beetroot
½ cup carrots
2 mint leaves
½ cup spinach
2 Tablespoons of chia seeds

Lunch: Vegetable Salad Raw OR Lightly Steamed
1 cup of chopped or shredded Brussels sprouts
½ cup sweet potatoes (cooked)
½ cup of snow peas
½ cup cauliflower
Take ½ lemon and sprinkle over vegetables

Snack: ½ cup blueberries

Dinner: Vegetable Stew

Instructions: In a large saucepan, sauté onions and garlic. Then add your favorite veggies, sauté for another 2 minutes. Add 2 cups of filtered water and sea salt to taste. Slow cook until veggies are done. You could blend the ingredients for a thick broth or eat it as is with chunks of veggies.

Snack: 8 oz of water and ½ grapefruit

End of the day reflections
How I felt today (1 lousy and 5 fantastic!)
Mood: 1 2 3 4 5
Energy: 1 2 3 4 5
Digestion: 1 2 3 4 5
Cravings: 1 2 3 4 5
Loving thought before bed:

Self-care check in:
- ❏ morning intentions
- ❏ home-cooked food
- ❏ mindful eating
- ❏ laughter
- ❏ time to myself
- ❏ spoke my purpose out loud
- ❏ prayer/meditation
- ❏ fresh air
- ❏ meaningful interactions
- ❏ conscious breathing
- ❏ intentional movement

Day 2

Morning detox water: 1 full cup (8 oz) of warm water with ½ of a lemon

Morning meditation and deep breathing:
What are your intentions for today?

What is your water intake goal for today?

Sleep:
Describe your sleeping conditions (lighting, noise, interruptions, etc)

What was the quality of your sleep?

Breakfast: Green Smoothie
1 kiwi
1 small apple
¼ cup pineapple
2 celery stalks
2 cups spinach
1 cup water

Lunch: Asparagus Salad
8 asparagus Spears
1 tsp of olive oil
½ cup of tomatoes
1 teaspoons of fresh herbs

Instructions: Steam asparagus for about 2-4 minute. Cool in ice bath. Dry. Add tomatoes and fresh herbs. Enjoy!

Snack: 1 cup of organic green tea

Dinner: 1 small baked sweet potato 1 cup of steamed broccoli, 1 cup of chopped beats, steamed with 2 teaspoons of avocado dressing*

*Instructions for dressing: 1 ripe avocado, 1 teaspoon of apple cider vinegar, ¼ teaspoon of garlic powder, 4 teaspoons of water.

Snack: 8 oz of water and 1 small orange

End of the day reflections
How I felt today (1 lousy to 5 fantastic!)
Mood: 1 2 3 4 5
Energy: 1 2 3 4 5
Digestion: 1 2 3 4 5
Cravings: 1 2 3 4 5

What joy did your day bring?

What obstacles did you face?

Loving thought before bed:

Self-care check in:

- ❏ morning intentions
- ❏ home-cooked food
- ❏ mindful eating
- ❏ laughter
- ❏ time to myself
- ❏ spoke my purpose out loud
- ❏ prayer/meditation
- ❏ fresh air
- ❏ meaningful interactions
- ❏ conscious breathing
- ❏ intentional movement

Day 3

Morning detox water: 1 full cup (8 oz) of warm water with ½ of a lemon

Morning meditation and deep breathing:
What are your intentions for today?

What is your water intake goal for today?

Breakfast Fruit Bowl
¼ cup of blueberries
1 teaspoons of flaxseed ground
½ cup of cantaloupe, seeded

Instructions: Mix berries and flaxseed. Spoon in cantaloupe

Lunch: Chickpea Salad
1 cup of chickpeas
1 small red onion
1 celery stalk
1 red pepper
1 garlic clove
¼ cup of lemon juice

½ teaspoon
½ teaspoon of sea salt

Instructions: Combine all ingredients in a large bowl and toss well. Let sit for about 30 minutes to let the flavors mingle. Then enjoy.

Snack: 1 cup of organic green tea

Dinner: Hearty Bowl
½ cup cooked quinoa
1 cup of steamed vegetables
1 cup of kale or spinach
2 teaspoons of olive oil
1 teaspoon of lemon juice
½ avocado sliced
Black pepper to taste

Instructions: Add quinoa to the bottom of the bowl. Top with vegetables and a handful of spinach or kale. Dress lightly with olive oil and lemon. Top with avocado

Snack: 8 oz of water with lemon

End of the day reflections
How I felt today (1 lousy and 5 fantastic!)
Mood: 1 2 3 4 5
Energy: 1 2 3 4 5
Digestion: 1 2 3 4 5
Cravings: 1 2 3 4 5

How do you feel?

What are you going to do to move one step closer to becoming a healthier and happier you?

Loving thought before bed:

Self-care check in:

❏ morning intentions   ❏ prayer/meditation
❏ home-cooked food   ❏ fresh air
❏ mindful eating   ❏ meaningful interactions
❏ laughter   ❏ conscious breathing
❏ time to myself   ❏ intentional movement
❏ spoke my purpose out loud

Day 4

Morning detox water: 1 full cup (8 oz) of warm water with ½ of a lemon

Morning meditation and deep breathing:
What are your intentions for today?

What is your water intake goal for today?

My body feels _____
My mind feels _____
My emotions are _____
My spirit is _____

Breakfast: Carrot Apple Celery Juice Make in Juicer
2 large carrots
1 apple
2 celery stalks
Ice optional
Blend and enjoy

Lunch: Cucumber and Tomato Salad

1 cup of chopped and peeled cucumber
½ cup of cherry tomato
1 green bell pepper
¼ cup of red onion
¼ cup of fresh or ground herbs
3 tablespoons of olive oil
1 tablespoon of red wine vinegar

Instructions: Place cucumbers, cherry tomatoes, red onion and green pepper into a large bowl. Make the dressing. Pour over the vegetables. Toss to coat. Enjoy

Snack: 1 cup of organic green tea

Dinner: black beans, curry cauliflower and sweet potato plate
1 cup of organic black beans rinsed
1 cup of roasted cauliflower
1 cup of cubed roasted sweet potatoes
¼ cup of curry powder

Instructions: Pour 2 tablespoons of olive oil over the cauliflower and sweet potatoes and Roast the sweet potatoes and cauliflower for about 30 minutes in 400-degree oven. Once done and cooled, place the black beans, heated, into a bowl. Add the cauliflower and sweet potato on top. Enjoy

Snack 8 oz of water with lemon

End of the day reflections
How I felt today (1 lousy and 5 fantastic!)
Mood: 1 2 3 4 5
Energy: 1 2 3 4 5
Digestion: 1 2 3 4 5
Cravings: 1 2 3 4 5

Reflect on your physical body as it exists now. What do you love most about your body? What areas would you like to improve?

Loving thought before bed:

Self-care check in:
- ❏ morning intentions
- ❏ home-cooked food
- ❏ mindful eating
- ❏ laughter
- ❏ time to myself
- ❏ spoke my purpose out loud
- ❏ prayer/meditation
- ❏ fresh air
- ❏ meaningful interactions
- ❏ conscious breathing
- ❏ intentional movement

Day 5

Morning detox water: 1 full cup (8 oz) of warm water with ½ of a lemon

Morning meditation and deep breathing:
What are your intentions for today?
What is your water intake goal for today?

What time did you wake up?
How many hours did you sleep?
Was your sleep interrupted? If so, what woke you up?

Breakfast: tofu scramble
8 ounces firm tofu
¼ tsp salt
¼ tsp turmeric powder
1/8 tsp ground black pepper

Instructions: Chop the tofu and use a fork to crumble it into bite-sized pieces. Add some water or oil to a frying pan and when it's hot, add the tofu and the rest of the ingredients. Stir until well combined and cook over medium-high heat for 5 to 10 minutes. Stir occasionally. Serve tofu scramble with fresh parsley.

Lunch: Mango spinach salad
1 cup of spinach one half cup of tomatoes 4 avocado slices
1 ounce of pecans one fourth cup of mango
2 tablespoons of olive oil and one-half lemon as dressing.

Snack: 8 oz of organic green tea

Dinner: Beet Soup
 1 small red onion diced
 1 ½ pounds beets trimmed and cut into 1/2-inch cubes
 (about 4 cups)
 1 tablespoon finely minced ginger root
 2 garlic cloves minced
 2 cups water or vegetable stock
 1 teaspoon sea salt
 1 cup whole raw cashews
 2 tablespoons lime juice plus 1 whole lime cut into
 wedges for garnish
 ¼ cup cilantro leaves for garnish

Instructions

In a large stockpot or Dutch oven, heat the oil over medium-high heat. Sauté the onion until translucent and soft, 5 minutes. Add the beets, ginger, and garlic. Cook for 5 more minutes, or until vibrant in color and quite fragrant

Carefully pour stock and salt into the pan, scraping up any brown bits that may have formed. Bring to a simmer, cover, and cook until the beets are tender, 35 to 40 minutes. During the last 15 minutes of cooking, stir in the cashews

Off the heat, stir in the lime juice and taste for seasoning. Puree until very smooth with an immersion blender or in a high-powered stand blender

Divide between 4 bowls and garnish with the cilantro leaves and a few lime wedges

Snack 8ounces of water with lemon

End of the day reflections
How I felt today (1 lousy and 5 fantastic!)
Mood: 1 2 3 4 5
Energy: 1 2 3 4 5
Digestion: 1 2 3 4 5
Cravings: 1 2 3 4 5

How can you love yourself better today?

What does it mean to be your highest self?

Loving thought before bed:

Self-care check in:
❏ morning intentions   ❏ prayer/meditation
❏ home-cooked food   ❏ fresh air
❏ mindful eating   ❏ meaningful interactions
❏ laughter   ❏ conscious breathing
❏ time to myself   ❏ intentional movement

❏ spoke my purpose out loud

Day 6

Morning detox water: 1 full cup (8 oz) of warm water with ½ of a lemon

Morning meditation and deep breathing:
What are your intentions for today?

What is your water intake goal for today?

What time did you wake up?

Breakfast: Beet and Apple Juice
1 medium beet
1 small apple
½ of lemon
Juice and enjoy

Snack: 1 cup of melon and 1 cup of green tea

Lunch: Vegetable and Amaranth Plate
1 small sweet potato
8 grilled asparagus spears
½ cup of amaranth
½ avocado
½ cup of zucchini

Cook amaranth according to the directions. Heat a skillet with 1 tablespoon of olive oil. Grill the asparagus until tender about 2-3 minutes on each side. Place ½ cup of amaranth onto plate. Add vegetables and add fresh herbs to top.

Dinner: Rainbow Rollups
4 collard green leaves
1 cup of shredded carrots
1 cup of shredded red cabbage
1 cup of cucumbers cut into match sticks
Juice of a lime
4 tablespoons of organic hummus

Instructions: Take one cleaned and dried collard green leaf. Spread 1 tablespoon of organic humus on the leaf. Add shredded carrots, cabbage and cucumbers. Repeat until all 4 rollups are made. Enjoy!

Snack: 8 oz of water with lemon

End of the day reflection
How I felt today (1 lousy and 5 fantastic!)
Mood: 1 2 3 4 5
Energy: 1 2 3 4 5
Digestion: 1 2 3 4 5
Cravings: 1 2 3 4 5

What is your ideal life?

What can you do to start living your ideal life?

Loving thought before bed:

Self-care check in:
❏ morning intentions   ❏ prayer/meditation

❑ home-cooked food   ❑ fresh air
❑ mindful eating   ❑ meaningful interactions
❑ laughter   ❑ conscious breathing
❑ time to myself   ❑ intentional movement
❑ spoke my purpose out loud

Day 7

Morning detox water: 1 full cup (8 oz) of warm water with ½ of a lemon.

Morning meditation and deep breathing:
What are your intentions for today?

What is your water intake goal for today?

Breakfast:
1 grapefruit
1 ounce of raw walnuts

Snack: 8 oz of green tea

Lunch: Curry cauliflower and sweet potato bowl
1 medium to large cauliflower cut and cleaned
2-3 tablespoons of curry
1 teaspoon of Himalayan salt
2 tablespoons of olive oil
2-3 sweet potatoes cleaned and cut
1 cup of cooked quinoa
Large sheet pan

Instructions: Pre heat oven to 425 degrees Fahrenheit. Clean and cut cauliflower. Pat completely dry. Peel and cut sweet potatoes into equal ½ inch rounds. Cut each sweet potato round into ½ inch equal sized pieces

● ● ●

Add cauliflower, sweet potatoes, olive oil, salt and curry into a bowl. Mix together

Place onto a large nonstick sheet pan. Toss every 10-15 minutes until tender about 20-30 minutes

Prepare quinoa according to the package directions. Serve over cooked quinoa and fresh parsley

Dinner: Detox Crockpot Lentil Soup
2 cups butternut squash (peeled and cubed)
2 cups carrots (peeled and sliced)
2 cups potatoes (chopped)
2 cups celery (chopped)
1 cup green lentils
3/4 cup yellow split peas (or just use more lentils)
1 onion (chopped)
5 cloves garlic (minced)
8–10 cups vegetable or chicken broth
2 teaspoons herbs de provence
1 teaspoon salt (more to taste)

ADD AT THE END:
2–3 cups kale (stems removed, chopped)
1 cup parsley (chopped)
½ cup olive oil – rosemary olive oil or other herb infused oil is delicious
a swish of sherry, red wine vinegar, or lemon juice to add a nice tangy bite

Snack: 8 oz of water with cucumber

The Halfway Point!
Visualizing My Future

Right about now is when so many people lose steam, focus or discipline to get past the halfway point. This is a reminder that you came to finish this race! My mother always said, "Start with the end in mind!" Take a minute to remind yourself why you are making this lifelong change to becoming a healthier and happier version of yourself. **Visualization exercise:**

Close your eyes and picture yourself 5 years from now. Allow yourself to meditate on this vision for 10 minutes then open your eyes and answer these questions.

What are you doing?

Where are you living?

Who is in your life?

What is important to you?

What have you achieved and experienced?
Now it's time to manifest that life…keep going!

Day 8

Morning detox water: 1 full cup (8 oz) of warm water with ½ of a lemon.

Morning meditation and deep breathing:
What are your intentions for today?

What is your water intake goal for today?

Breakfast: Citrus Fruit Salad with pecans
½ cup of blueberries
½ cup of strawberries
½ cup of pears
½ of a lemon
1 ounce of unroasted unsalted pecans
Instructions: Place fruit in a bowl. Sprinkle with fresh lemon juice. Add pecans. Enjoy.

Snack: ½ of avocado and 5 carrot sticks

Lunch: Grilled tomato and broccoli salad
2 large tomatoes sliced in rounds
1 medium whole fresh broccoli
2 tablespoons of olive oil
⅓ teaspoon of Italian seasoning
2 cups of spinach
2 tablespoons of balsamic vinegar
Heat olive oil in a grill pan. Take sliced tomatoes and top with Italian seasoning.

Place on grill pan for 2-3 minutes on each side. Once tender, place on a plate and let cool. Clean spinach and broccoli. Cut broccoli into bite sized pieces.

Take the spinach and put into a bowl. Add tomatoes and broccoli. Add balsamic vinegar. Enjoy!

Dinner: Quinoa sautéed spinach and sweet potato plate
2 cups of cooked quinoa
2 cups of spinach
1 cup sweet potatoes
2 tablespoons of olive oil
1 teaspoon of Himalayan salt

Instructions: Prepare quinoa according to package directions. Roast sweet potatoes in a 400-degree F oven for about 30 minutes turning frequently. Place 1 tablespoon of olive oil into a pan. Add spinach and saute until tender. Place on a plate. Add quinoa and sweet potatoes. Enjoy!

Snack: 1 cup of green tea unsweetened

End of the day reflection
How I felt today (1 lousy and 5 fantastic!)
Mood: 1 2 3 4 5
Energy: 1 2 3 4 5
Digestion: 1 2 3 4 5
Cravings: 1 2 3 4 5

Are you living an authentic life? What steps will you take to help you live true to yourself?

Loving thought before bed:

Self-care check in:
❑ morning intentions   ❑ prayer/meditation
❑ home-cooked food   ❑ fresh air
❑ mindful eating   ❑ meaningful interactions
❑ laughter   ❑ conscious breathing
❑ time to myself   ❑ intentional movement
❑ spoke my purpose out loud

Day 9

Morning detox water: 1 full cup (8 oz) of warm water with ½ of a lemon

Morning meditation and deep breathing:
What are your intentions for today?

What is your water intake goal for today?

Breakfast: Green Smoothie Make in Juicer add ice as an option
1 kiwi
1 small apple
¼ cup pineapple
2 celery stalks
2 cups spinach
1 cup water

Snack: 1 cup of green tea

Lunch: Spinach salad
1 large bag of organic spinach
1 cup of cherry tomatoes sliced
½ cup of walnuts chopped
½ cup of cooked amaranth
½ cup of yellow and red peppers mixed cleaned and diced into small pieces
3 tablespoons of olive oil
3 tablespoons of red wine vinegar

Instructions: In a large bowl, place spinach, tomatoes, walnuts, peppers, olive oil and red wine vinegar into a bowl. Mix well. Serve. Add an additional tablespoon of red wine vinegar of salad is too dry.

Dinner: Summer squash soup
1 tablespoon of olive oil

½. cup minced yellow onion
2 cups finely diced yellow summer squash
¼ cup diced carrot
1 clove garlic minced
¾ teaspoon cumin powder
½ teaspoon coriander
½ teaspoon turmeric
½ teaspoon paprika
¼ teaspoon cinnamon
pinch cayenne pepper optional
2 cups low-sodium vegetable broth
¼ cup coconut water
Salt to taste
Cilantro for topping
Dollop of organic yogurt

Instructions: Heat a heavy-bottomed pot over medium-low heat. Add the olive oil followed by the onions. Cook until the onions are fragrant and translucent, 4 to 5 minutes. Stir in the squash, and carrot.

Continue to cook for until the squash begins to soften, 5 minutes or so. Stir in the garlic, cook for a minute then add in all the spices, cooking for another minute more. Add in the vegetable broth. Bring to a boil, reduce to a simmer, and let cook 10 to 15 minutes.

Puree the soup using a blender or an immersion blender. Add in the coconut water and continue to heat the soup until hot. Taste and add salt as needed (usually depends on how salty the broth is). Divide into two bowls and top with yogurt, sprinkle of paprika, and cilantro.

Snack: 8 oz of water and small apple
End of the day reflection
How I felt today (1 lousy and 5 fantastic!)

Mood: 1 2 3 4 5
Energy: 1 2 3 4 5
Digestion: 1 2 3 4 5
Cravings: 1 2 3 4 5

What bad habits do you want to break?

What good habits do you want to cultivate?

Loving thought before bed:

Self-care check in:
❏ morning intentions   ❏ prayer/meditation
❏ home-cooked food   ❏ fresh air
❏ mindful eating   ❏ meaningful interactions
❏ laughter   ❏ conscious breathing
❏ time to myself   ❏ intentional movement
❏ spoke my purpose out loud

Day 10

Morning detox water: 1 full cup (8 oz) of warm water with ½ of lemon

Morning meditation and deep breathing:
What are your intentions for today?

What is your water intake goal for today?
Breakfast: Hot Quinoa Bowl with Almonds and Blueberries

2 cups of water
1 cup of quinoa ⅛ teaspoon of cinnamon
½ cup of blueberries.
1 ounce of plain unsalted unroasted almonds

Instructions: Bring water to a boil. Add quinoa. Return to
a boil. Reduce heat, cover and simmer about 10-15
minutes. Add cinnamon. Let cool. Add blueberries. Enjoy.

Snack ½ of Avocado and ½ red bell pepper

Lunch: Balsamic Vinegar Roasted Vegetables

Dinner: Spaghetti Squash and Tomato Salad
1 large spaghetti squash cut in half and cooked
1 cup of cherry tomatoes sliced
½ cup of chopped cucumber
1 teaspoons of sea salt
1 small red onion
½ cup of red wine vinegar

Instructions: Preheat oven to 350 degrees Fahrenheit. Cut
spaghetti squash in half and clean all the seeds. Place on a
large baking sheet with the skin up.

Cook for about 60 minutes or until tender. Once cooled
scrape the content of the spaghetti squash out into a bowl
with a fork.

Place chopped tomatoes, cucumbers, red onion and salt into
a separate bowl. Add vinegar and mix together. Serve the
squash and salad on a plate. Enjoy.

Snack 8 oz of green tea
End of the day reflections
How I felt today (1 lousy and 5 fantastic!)

Mood: 1 2 3 4 5
Energy: 1 2 3 4 5
Digestion: 1 2 3 4 5
Cravings: 1 2 3 4 5

What is your internal dialogue like? Is it filled with positive or negative self-talk?

What limiting beliefs are you holding on to?

Loving thought before bed:

Self-care check in:
- ❏ morning intentions
- ❏ home-cooked food
- ❏ mindful eating
- ❏ laughter
- ❏ time to myself
- ❏ spoke my purpose out loud
- ❏ prayer/meditation
- ❏ fresh air
- ❏ meaningful interactions
- ❏ conscious breathing
- ❏ intentional movement

Day 11

Morning detox water: 1 full cup (8 oz) of warm water with ½ of a lemon

Morning meditation and deep breathing:
What are your intentions for today?

What is your water intake goal for today?

Breakfast: Cranberry and Apple Juice
1 ½ cups cranberries
1 apple
3 celery stalks
3 leaves of romaine lettuce
½ thumb of ginger
½ lemon, peeled

Instructions: Place all of the ingredients through a juicer and enjoy!

Lunch: Grilled Vegetable Lettuce Wraps

Snack: 1 cup of green tea

Dinner: Mizuna, Fennel, and Mulberry Salad
1 large fennel bulb, including fronds
1 large bunch mizuna, stems trimmed and removed
¼ cup chopped fresh parsley
2 tablespoons fresh lemon juice
2 tablespoons olive oil
1 ½ tablespoons fennel seeds
½ teaspoon sea salt
½ teaspoon freshly cracked black pepper, or more to taste
2/3 cup dried mulberries

Instructions: Trim off the fennel root and fronds, leaving a 1-inch handle on top of the bulb. Reserve the fronds. Use a mandolin to carefully shave the fennel bulb into paper-thin slices, yielding around 6 cups. Fill a bowl with an ice bath and place the fennel inside for about 10 minutes to crisp. In a small bowl, whisk together the lemon juice, olive oil, fennel seeds, sea salt and black pepper.

When the fennel is crisp, remove the shavings from the ice bath and drain thoroughly. Gently pat dry with towels to remove any excess moisture, and place in a large bowl along with the mizuna, parsley, and ⅓ cup mulberries. Toss to combine, add the dressing, and gently toss by hand to distribute the ingredients evenly. To serve, place in serving bowls, top with remaining mulberries and a few small sprigs of the reserved fennel fronds. Add additional black pepper if desired

End of the day reflections
How I felt today:
Mood: 1 2 3 4 5
Energy: 1 2 3 4 5
Digestion: 1 2 3 4 5
Cravings: 1 2 3 4 5

What would you want to say to yourself 1 year in the future?

Loving thought before bed:

Self-care check in:
❏ morning intentions   ❏ prayer/meditation
❏ home-cooked food   ❏ fresh air
❏ mindful eating   ❏ meaningful interactions
❏ laughter   ❏ conscious breathing
❏ time to myself   ❏ intentional movement
❏ spoke my purpose out loud

Day 12

Morning detox water: 1 full cup (8 oz) of warm water with ½ of a lemon

Morning meditation and deep breathing:

What are your intentions for today?

What is your water intake goal for today?

Breakfast: Tofu scramble
8 ounces firm tofu (225 g)
¼ tsp salt, see notes
¼ tsp turmeric powder, see notes
1/8 tsp ground black pepper

Instructions: Chop the tofu and use a fork to crumble it into bite-sized pieces. Add some water or oil to a frying pan and when it's hot, add the tofu and the rest of the ingredients. Stir until well combined and cook over medium-high heat for 5 to 10 minutes. Stir occasionally.

Snack: 1 cup of green tea with ½ cup of melon

Lunch: Detox Crockpot Lentil Soup

Dinner: Sweet Potato Hash with Grilled Vegetables
1–2 tbsp extra virgin olive oil
1 pound sweet potatoes, cubed
2 cloves of garlic, chopped
½ red onion, chopped
½ red bell pepper, chopped
½ green bell pepper, chopped
½ tsp salt
¼ tsp ground black pepper

*Use the recipe for the balsamic grilled vegetables from day 10.

Instructions: Heat the oil in a skillet, add the sweet potato cubes, cover with a lid and cook over medium heat for about 10 minutes, stirring occasionally. You don't have to peel the sweet potatoes, but it's up to you.

Add all the remaining ingredients, stir and cook uncovered over medium-high heat for about 10 to 15 minutes or until tender and golden brown.

Serve immediately (I added some chopped fresh parsley on top) or keep leftovers in an airtight container in the fridge for 3-5 days.

Snack 8 oz of water

End of the day reflections
How I felt today:
Mood: 1 2 3 4 5
Energy: 1 2 3 4 5
Digestion: 1 2 3 4 5
Cravings: 1 2 3 4 5

What fears are immobilizing you? Why?

Loving thought before bed:

Self-care check in:
❏ morning intentions   ❏ prayer/meditation
❏ home-cooked food   ❏ fresh air
❏ mindful eating   ❏ meaningful interactions
❏ laughter   ❏ conscious breathing
❏ time to myself   ❏ intentional movement
❏ spoke my purpose out loud

Day 13

Morning detox water: 1 full cup (8 oz) of warm water with ½ of a lemon

Morning meditation and deep breathing:
What are your intentions for today?

What is your water intake goal for today?

What time did you wake up?

Breakfast: Fig and Pear Salad
2 Figs halved
1 small pear sliced and diced
1 teaspoon of dried coconut.
1 ounce of unsalted raw macadamia bites.

Instructions: Place figs on a plate. Mix pear and nuts in a bowl. Add to the plate. Sprinkle the coconut on top. Enjoy.

Snack: 8 oz of green tea with ½ grapefruit

Lunch: Vegan Veggie Burger with Butter Lettuce Top
¼ cup ground flax
½ cup water
3 cups cooked black beans (2 15-oz cans, drained and rinsed)
1 cup cashews* optional
1 ½ cups cooked brown rice
½ cup chopped parsley
1 ½ cups shredded carrots
1/3 cup chopped green onions
1 cup breadcrumbs* optional
2 tablespoons smoked paprika
1 tablespoon chili powder
1-2 teaspoons salt, to taste

Instructions: In a small bowl, combine the ground flax and water. Give it a little stir and set aside. In a large bowl, add the drained and rinsed black beans. Mash with a potato masher (or fork) until most of the beans are a paste. Leave about ¼ of the beans whole.

Place the cashews in a food processor, and pulse until they are breadcrumb size, NOT a powder. It's okay if a few larger pieces remain. Add to the bowl with the beans. Now add the flax/water mix and all the remaining ingredients. Mix very well with a large wooden spoon. Using about 1/2 cup per burger, shape into burger patty shapes about 3/4 inch thick.

Preheat the oven to 350 degrees Farenheit and line a baking sheet or two with parchment paper. Place the patties on the pan(s) and bake for 20 minutes. Flip bake for 15 more minutes. Remove from oven.

Serve with 1 large butter lettuce leaf. Enjoy.

Snack: 8 oz of green tea with 1-2 cup of strawberries

Dinner: Tomato Basil Soup
3 pounds ripe plum tomatoes, cut in half lengthwise
¼ cup plus 2 tablespoons good olive oil
1 tablespoon kosher salt
1 ½ teaspoons freshly ground black pepper
2 cups chopped yellow onions (2 onions)
6 garlic cloves, minced
2 tablespoons unsalted butter
¼ teaspoon crushed red pepper flakes
1 (28-ounce) canned plum tomatoes, with their juice
4 cups fresh basil leaves, packed
1 teaspoon fresh thyme leaves
1 quart chicken stock or water

Instructions: Preheat the oven to 400 degrees F. Toss together the tomatoes, 1/4 cup olive oil, salt, and pepper. Spread the tomatoes in 1 layer on a baking sheet and roast for 45 minutes.

In an 8-quart stockpot over medium heat, saute the onions and garlic with 2 tablespoons of olive oil, the butter, and red pepper flakes for 10 minutes, until the onions start to brown. Add the canned tomatoes, basil, thyme, and chicken stock. Add the oven-roasted tomatoes, including the liquid on the baking sheet. Bring to a boil and simmer uncovered for 40 minutes. Pass through a food mill fitted with the coarsest blade. Taste for seasonings. Serve hot or cold.

Snack: 8 oz of water

End of the day reflections
How I felt today (1 lousy and 5 fantastic!)
Mood: 1 2 3 4 5
Energy: 1 2 3 4 5
Digestion: 1 2 3 4 5
Cravings: 1 2 3 4 5

If you had a magic wand what wand you instantly change in your life and why?

Loving thought before bed:

Self-care check in:
❏ morning intentions   ❏ prayer/meditation
❏ home-cooked food   ❏ fresh air
❏ mindful eating   ❏ meaningful interactions
❏ laughter   ❏ conscious breathing
❏ time to myself   ❏ intentional movement

❑ spoke my purpose out loud

Day 14

Morning detox water: 1 full cup (8 oz) of warm water with ½ of a lemon

Morning meditation and deep breathing:
What are your intentions for today?

What is your water intake goal for today?

Breakfast: Raspberry Lemon, apple and spinach blended into a juice

Snack: 8 oz of green tea 5 carrots ½ avocado.

Lunch: Black Bean Soup

Dinner: Vegetable Plate
½ Avocado
6 carrot sticks
½ cup of chopped red peppers
4 radish cleaned and sliced
½ cup of cherry tomatoes

Place vegetables on a plate and enjoy.
Snack 8 oz of water

End of the day reflections
How I felt today (1 lousy and 5 fantastic!)
Mood: 1 2 3 4 5
Energy: 1 2 3 4 5
Digestion: 1 2 3 4 5
Cravings: 1 2 3 4 5

What are the biggest actions you can take now to create the biggest results in your life?

Where are you living right now – the past, future or present?

Are you living your life to the fullest right now?

Loving thought before bed:

Self-care check in:
- ❏ morning intentions
- ❏ home-cooked food
- ❏ mindful eating
- ❏ laughter
- ❏ time to myself
- ❏ spoke my purpose out loud
- ❏ prayer/meditation
- ❏ fresh air
- ❏ meaningful interactions
- ❏ conscious breathing
- ❏ intentional movement

Day 15

Morning detox water: 1 full cup (8 oz) of warm water with ½ of a lemon

Morning meditation and deep breathing:
What are your intentions for today?
What is your water intake goal for today?

Breakfast: ½ cup papaya with 1 ounce of raw walnuts

Snack: 8 oz of green tea with 2 celery sticks and ½ cup of cooked black beans

Lunch: Artichoke Salad
8 asparagus cooked, cleaned and chopped
½ cup of yellow cherry tomatoes sliced in halves
½ red onion chopped
½ cup of chick peas
3 tablespoons of olive oil
½ cucumber sliced and diced
¼ teaspoon of Italian seasoning
Juice of ½ lemon
¼ cup of your favorite vinegar
Fresh herbs to top
Salt and pepper to taste

Instructions: Place cooked asparagus, tomatoes, onions, chickpeas, cucumber in a bowl. Toss well. I'm a separate bowl, mix olive oil, vinegar and juice of the lemon together. Add salt and pepper to taste.

Pour over vegetables. Toss well. Top with fresh herbs. And enjoy!

Dinner: Brown Rice Vegetable Bowl
½ cup of mushroom
½ cup of mixed color peppers
½ cup of brown rice
½ onion
½ cup of spinach
3 tablespoons of olive oil
Salt and pepper to taste.
Fresh herbs to top
Instructions: Clean and dice mushrooms, onions, and peppers. In a large pan, sauté vegetables with olive oil until tender. Add spinach last masking sure to not over cook. Put to the side.

Take ½ cup of cooked brown rice and place in a bowl. Put vegetables on top and sprinkle with fresh herbs and salt and pepper to taste. Enjoy.

Snack: 8 oz of water with ½ cup blueberries.

End of the day reflections
How I felt today (1 lousy and 5 fantastic!)
Mood: 1 2 3 4 5
Energy: 1 2 3 4 5
Digestion: 1 2 3 4 5
Cravings: 1 2 3 4 5

What is the biggest change you've noticed within yourself?

Loving thought before bed:

Self-care check in:
❑ morning intentions   ❑ prayer/meditation
❑ home-cooked food   ❑ fresh air
❑ mindful eating   ❑ meaningful interactions
❑ laughter   ❑ conscious breathing
❑ time to myself   ❑ intentional movement
❑ spoke my purpose out loud

Life after the cleanse

What has changed for you?

What mindset shift did you experience?

What healthy commitments are you ready to make?

What are your long-term goals for your mental, physical, emotional and spiritual wellbeing?

How do you feel?

How much weight did you release?

Did you meet your weight goal?

Did you meet your emotional health goal?

What have you learned about yourself?

How are you going to keep this going?

What were your obstacles?

How will you overcome them?

References

Imparato, L. 2016. Healthy Solutions For Teal Life: RETOX Yoga, Food, Attitude. New York, Berkeley Books.

Crockpot Lentil Soup recipe courtesy of https://pinchofyum.com/the-best-detox-crockpot-lentil-soup

Beet Soup recipe courtesy of https://feedmephoebe.com/detox-red-beet-soup-recipe/

ABOUT THE AUTHOR

Jeanette received her Master of Science Degree in Family and Consumer Science from Bowling Green State University in December of 1997. She then went on to become a Registered Dietitian in 1999 where she began her career as the head dietitian at Deaton Hospital in Baltimore, MD. Jeanette challenged herself by trying different opportunities. She worked for the State of Maryland and for a food service company in Frederick, MD as a nutritionist. In 2000, Jeanette received a certificate in weight management from the American Dietetic Association. Shortly after, she joined the first ladies of football, the Washington Redskins Cheerleaders, where she spent four years entertaining, traveling the world and evolving into an athlete.

For the last 12 years, Jeanette has spent the majority of her career in the Pharmaceutical Industry where she continued to utilize her skills as a dietitian. Winning several awards including the prestigious President's Club twice, her passion for helping others inspired her to fulfill her dream of being an entrepreneur. After the birth of her son, Jeanette started *Fit With Jeanette Chandler*, a company geared toward helping women rediscover who they are through health and fitness. Her greatest accomplishment has been a wife to her husband and the mother of her amazing little boy. In her free time, Jeanette enjoys running, spending time with friends and reading.